DHANWANTARI

The secret to health is knowing how to deal with one's body. These life practices are not mystical or esoteric in nature, rather they deal with down-to-earth habits of daily living which can produce a tremendous improvement in mental and physical health. The practical daily habits dealt with in this book by Harish Johari include suggestions for regulating bowel habits, diet, sleep, meditation, water intake, sex, drug intake, breathing, massage, nostril and hemispheric predominance, planetary and lunar influences, and cyclic changes in our endocrine system. In this book, the reader will learn how to control these variables in human functioning which need regulations in order to achieve a balanced, happy and productive life.

How India's ancient art of living and healing
can give you a healthier, happier,
more joyous life

Dhanwantari

Harish Johari

with an introduction by
Michael Gerber, M.D.

Rupa & Co

First published by
Rams Head Inc., San Francisco, California

First in Rupa Paperback 1992
Eleventh Impression 2009

Published by

Rupa . Co

7/16, Ansari Road, Daryaganj
New Delhi 110 002

Sales Centres:

Allahabad Bengalooru Chandigarh Chennai
Hyderabad Jaipur Kathmandu
Kolkata Mumbai

ISBN 81-7167-101-2

Typeset in 10/12 pts Baskerville by
Mindways Design
1410 Chiranjiv Tower
43 Nehru Place
New Delhi 110 019

Printed in India by
Anubha Printers
B-48, Sector-7
Noida 201 301

Harish Johari

Harish Johari is a poet, artist, musician, teacher, farmer, philosopher, scholar and translator. He is also a physiologist, historian and expert cinematographer.

Johari was born in 1934 in Bareilly, Uttar Pradesh, in Northern India about eighty miles from the Nepal border. His father, a Yogi and Magistrate, taught the fundamental life habits necessary to attain the greatest development of the body and consciousness. It is the relationship between these daily living habits and their profound effect on the individual's energy level which Johari feels people need to learn in order to achieve normalcy, good health and a foundation for elevating consciousness.

Since childhood, Johari has been recognized as an extraordinarily gifted and creative person. His many talents and sincere desire for a correct understanding of the truth have attracted many teachers including saints, physicians, artists and important political and cultural figures of India. He has received two Master's degrees: one in Urdu Literature from Lucknow University, the other in Philosophy from Agra University.

Johari has also created many beautiful sculptures and paintings in the cities and temples of India and, in the process, developed revolutionary techniques in both media.

His books have been published in the English, Dutch, German and Spanish languages. Harish Johari has been travelling, teaching, presenting multistrata seminars about 'Living in Awareness' in Europe, Mexico and the U.S.A. He now lives with his family in Princeton, N.J., and Berkeley, California.

Contents

Introduction

The secret to health is knowing how to deal with one's body. These life practices are not mystical or esoteric in nature, rather they deal with down-to-earth habits of daily living which can produce a tremendous improvement in mental and physical health. The practical, daily habits dealt with in this book by Harish Johari include suggestions for regulating bowel habits, diet, sleep, meditation, water intake, sex, drug intake, breathing, massage, nostril and hemispheric predominance, planetary and lunar influences and cyclic changes in our endocrine system. In this book, the reader will learn how to control these variables in human functioning which need regulations in order to achieve a balanced, happy and productive life.

In 1966, along with Shyam Bhatnagar,* he established Satyam Shivam Sundaram, an institution to promote a synthesis of Eastern and Western knowledge, each culture adding its particular strengths toward the goal of greater understanding of the body and life. Two years later, Johari made his first trip to the United States and began teaching psychologists and therapists at the New School of Social Research in New York City about the effects of sound on consciousness. He has lived and travelled with notable persons from both India and America throughout these years and talked with many American scholars and spiritual seekers. In the process, he enjoyed the good heart and openness of the American people, but at the same time discovered that Americans, in general, had very little practical knowledge about

---

* Psychotherapist and lifelong friend and student of Harish Johari.*

keeping their bodies functioning efficiently. During these travels, he also began collecting scientific data generated by Western technology which corroborates the validity of his ancient living habits. In 1972 he returned to the United States and, with the aid of Tariq Hamid, a psychotherapist, Sufi and cosmologist interested in East-West synthesis, established the Tantra Research Institute* (TRI) in Oakland, California.

As a physician, I find knowledge of these life habits of enormous benefit in treating patients and myself as well. It fills the gaps in my Western medical training which was not much concerned with these daily prac-ticalities. Unquestionably my patients and friends suf-fering poor mental or physical health heal more quickly when these energy-conserving life habits are included in treatment. This information gives every man the tools to cure a great majority of his problems without resorting to unnecessary drug therapy. When applied, this daily routine of attention to the body performed at home is far more effective in maintaining health (especially mental health) than intermittent clinical treatment. Our Western medical system (Allopathic system) responds only to mental and physical disease already present in the patient. But most diseases are caused by poor life habits, lack of a tailor-made diet for each individual, and uninformed drug intake across a span of years. Since these life habits are responsible for creating sickness, it is only logical that they must be dealt with in therapy if a lasting cure of body or psyche is expected. In these matters of daily practical importance, the Hindus and Tantrics have a much more sophisticated knowledge about the body and its control system than do we.

The first problem I see in my patients encountering these habits is that they don't understand how good it

---

* Tantra — comes from 'Tanuvistare', to spread out. Specifically, it refers to the spreading out of energy through the human system.

feels to be normal. The hyperstimulating American lifestyle of heavy meat intake, alcohol and coffee consumption, disregard of daily body rhythms, over-eating, no prayer or meditation, constipation, too frequent and short duration of sex and speeded up, stressful living is producing an American highly prone to illness with no worthy goals and no examples of human excellence toward which to aspire. This state of affairs is, indeed, normal for many Americans but is quite different from the Hindu definition of normalcy. Their normal state of being occurs when one feels light, energetic, calm and inspired to do his work every day. To live in this kind of "normal" state is difficult to imagine for Americans who presently exist in states of chronic stress, fatigue, anger and insecurity. In this Hindu "normal" state, easily achievable by anyone, one experiences a constant enjoyment of living, feeling of clarity and openness and a great deal more available energy for work and creative projects. The difference is very remarkable.

In many areas of scientific research in the West (including my own area of research in Neuroendocrinology and Psychopharmacology), this ancient Sanskrit knowledge is proving to be compatible with the most recent, contemporary medical research findings. For example, the existence of the pineal gland and its functional relationship to light has been clearly established by research in the West for the past ten years. The pineal gland has long been identified by Yogis in India as the sixth *Chakra*, called *Ajna Chakra* or "The Third Eye." They found the pineal to be a powerful behaviour modifier, capable of slowing down the organism and balancing the activity of the hemispheres (two sides of the brain). Neuroendocrine (brain hormone) research has shown that the newly discovered hormone, melatonin, formed only in the pineal gland, is stimulated by darkness and by particular neurochemicals and drugs. Melatonin acts through a complex chemical pathway which decreases the levels of six (or seven) anterior pituitary hormones in the brain and literally slows down the body hormonally. Melatonin is involved with sex and sexual development, growth hormone levels, thyroid hormone levels, adrenal hormone levels and several of the body's diurnal (daily) cycles. This knowledge, just being discovered in the West, has been used practically as a body control system by Yogis for thousands of years in India. The pineal body will undoubtedly play an important role in Western psychiatry and medicine as techniques of pineal manipulation and their neurochemical bases are disseminated and understood.

Another important contribution of Johari's work is the recent recognition by medical scholars of striking similarities between Yogic knowledge and recent medical research studying lymphatic systems.* Hindus have used massage and pressure point manipulation for centuries dealing with specific points over lymph chains and lymph nodes without knowledge of their actual physical existence. Only in recent years has modern lymphangiography (dye and X-ray techniques) demonstrated the exact location of these tiny structures in the body. Amazingly, a chart of the ancient Hindu pressure points is nearly identical to a chart of the lymph system as identified by modern lymphangiography.

In addition to the pineal and lymph, the nature of our split brain (twin hemispheres) has recently attracted the attention of many medical researchers. Ornstein and others have found that the left hemisphere is concerned with more verbal and intellectual activities and that the right hemisphere is better able to handle visual and creative work. The science of *Swar Yoga* has applied this knowledge of the hemisphere of the brain for centuries

---

* Lymph is a clear fluid leaked out of capillaries which carries large molecules and bacteria to local lymph cleaning stations (lymph nodes) and contains essential body chemicals and large numbers of white blood cells.

and has determined the specific functions of each hemisphere.

They also noted a relationship between hemisphere and nostril functioning. These Yogis, through their experimentation, discovered that only one nostril functions at a time and that, without intervention, it changes about once an hour. To change one's nostril mechanically one need only lie down on his side, place a pillow under the rib cage and armpit and let the mucous in the nose move downwards for several minutes and open the upper nostril. They found that the open right nostril causes the left hemisphere to predominate and vice-versa. So by controlling the nostril which is open, the hemispheres of the brain can be regulated.

I find controlling the nostrils to be an invaluable asset to my life. The pleasure of eating (right nostril) defecation (right), showering (right), sex (males right and females left), drinking (left) and urinating (left) is markedly enhanced by controlling the proper nostril. Proper coordination of nostrils (hemispheres) with life functions saves energy and allows one to harmonize with these daily activities. After working at controlling your nostrils for a short time, it becomes so basic that you wonder how you survived without knowledge of it. One needs this information regarding nostril control of the brain in insure best sexual enjoyment, proper digestion and pleasurable elimination.

Hindu Yogis have long espoused the belief that the seat of wisdom in the body resides in the stomach. Further they have followed a vegetarian diet believing that the seat of wisdom should not be hyperstimulated by such foods as meat. Recent scientific work by Fernstrom and Wortman at M.I.T.* has demonstrated the subtle biochemical mechanism which causes a high protein diet to decrease levels of serotonin (low levels of serotonin are found in depressed humans) and

---

* M.I.T. — Scientific American, February 1974.

conversely, high carbohydrate diet (vegetarian diet) increases serotonin. This work is the first to demonstrate a dietary link with mental health and adds to the evidence in favour of becoming vegetarian. Practically speaking, as one begins to eliminate meat from his diet he feels more energetic, less nervous and less pressured. Additionally one ceases to need a deodorant (a daily bath or shower should suffice) and finds the smell of the stool to be much less offensive.

In regard to sex, it is important to note that by practising the life habits in this book, sexual power and control is markedly enhanced. Our country, which glorifies youth and sex, will find a new level of sophistication and fulfilment in the male-female relationship by following these life habits. Tantric sexual practices, especially, require this kind of normalcy and body purity to achieve very high and extended sexual experiences.

Americans find discussion of bowel habits and feces in general to be rather culturally taboo. The resultant ignorance about elimination has produced one of America's greatest areas of health naivete. Proper daily elimination is vitally necessary for the mental health of every man on this planet. Also, self-diagnosis by noting form and colour of stool is simple, useful knowledge for everybody. The greatest problem in elimination for Americans is constipation and late defecation. For example, it is common to treat patients who have bowel movements only once every 2 or 3 days. These people are told that this bowel pattern is within the normal range by their doctors who, simultaneously, treat their neurotic complaints, anxiety and depression with tranquillizers, antidepressants and inconsistent dietary suggestions. The basic problem of constipation and how to relieve it is not seriously dealt with in our system of health. Is it any wonder so many Americans are "up tight," to use the colloquialism.

There are several studies which propose explanations for this association of constipation with poor mental health. One of these comes from Japanese investigators who have recently found the hallucinogenic chemical dimethyltryptamine (DMT) in the urine of schizophrenics. Their evidence suggests that this abnormal chemical collects in genetically susceptible individuals after large amounts of tryptamine (parent amino acid to DMT) is produced by bacteria in the colon when the individual is constipated and the bacteria cannot be eliminated. Practically speaking, great improvement in the clinical appearance of acute schizophrenics (who are very constipated, often going for 3 to 4 weeks without a bowel movement) occurs when they first defecate and tend to relapse as they miss their daily bowel movement. Too many bowel movements per day is also harmful (over two) as excessive fecal production is caused by an abnormal hyperactivity of the gastrointestinal tract and is a sign of nervousness and poor digestion.

Among the daily living habits described by this book, perhaps the most significant is the dawn cycle. This book tells what to do to take advantage of the energy available at dawn.

The increase in energy and endurance which accompany early rising are quickly noticeable. Rising before dawn becomes the high point of the day when one learns how to tune in his mind and body to the powerful electrical and chemical events which occur at sunrise. Early rising causes one to be calm, centred, energetic and clear-headed. The differences in mood and endurance are striking.

The appearance of these daily habits and home remedies is very timely for Americans. In the United States there is a growing awareness that the responsibility for good health rests with the individual, his life habits, his diet and not with his doctor or medication. The first challenge for Americans is in learning how to slow down and become sensitive to their bodies.

It is also interesting to note the link between these health habits and the ones of our forefathers. Such notable books as Jethro Kloss's *Back to Eden* and Gunn's *Family Physician* provided practical medical knowledge for our own heritage of folk medicine. There is a remarkable similarity in daily habits and dietary suggestions found in these works and those presented in this book.

As you proceed to work on your own body, you will see the power and life implications which unfold from this knowledge. In the beginning, don't feel discouraged or think your body is too deteriorated to use these habits. They work for everyone and will increase one's energy on the first day. Use as much of the material as you can. This is not an all or nothing book. The effects are additive. Be patient with yourself. Changing these most rudimentary life habits takes a little time, and as we begin to increase our awareness it becomes clear that there is nothing more important in life than daily concern for one's body.

It is of great importance that the large majority of these principles have already been supported by scientific data. In search of truth, this East-West synthesis of health knowledge will continue to undergo scientific scrutiny so that the most effective techniques from both cultures can be used for preventing our unique American spectrum of mental and physical disease. Harish Johari's goal in initiating this synthesis is to give Americans who desire to improve their bodies and minds enough basic information to insure good health and make possible a greatly expanded breadth of life experiences.

Michael Gerber, M.D.
Palo Alto, California

Preface

This is a book for anyone who is seeking a logical, scientific and practically tested set of principles for daily life. It is a book about waking up, cleansing, eating, drinking, massage, sex and home remedies.

It is a book about right living, about synchronizing the individual organism with the cycles of the Cosmos which has given him birth. It is a book about becoming normal.

There are chapters on meditation, exercises and the cycle of breath — for, all these are ways of tuning the system in shorter spans of time. But this is not a book about getting high. It is a book about becoming right. As much as one goes high, so much he has to go low. This is a fundamental law of Universe, readily apparent from the practical experience of life.

This is a book about techniques of centring, about stabilizing one's energy, about creating a place within one's own being to which he can return at will. One who has a centre within himself can then look with detachment upon the ever-changing face of the illusory world. And he can even begin to laugh.

This book is based upon my own cultural experience and the ageless traditions of India. On the pages which follow are practices from *Yoga*, from *Ayurvedic* medicine (a system dating back thousands of years before Christ), from the ancient *Yunani* system of the Greeks and Moslems, and from the timeless tribal cultures which people the plains, deserts and mountains of the Indian subcontinent.

But the validity of these practices is not limited to

Indians. There is nothing on these pages which has not been tried successfully on and by those born and raised in America. Truth, to be worthy of its name, must be universal.

The bulk of this book springs directly from dictations given to a young Indian, Vinod Agarwal, and a young American, Dick Brenneman (who also assembled them into their present form). They, along with many others, implemented these practices in their own lives and found them worthy.

I am especially thankful to the psychologists, physiologists and experimental technicians of America for their tremendous work in developing and utilizing electronic instruments to detect and monitor the operation of the human organism. Their findings are remarkable, and an eye-opening experience for the Eastern-born thinker.

My visit to this country (America) has increased my respect and admiration for my own culture, who converted the mysteries of the play of body chemistry and the law of polarity and rhythm into religion. These same understandings Western science is now making known through its own avenues and approaches.

There is no conflict between ancient and modern knowledge. This much has become increasingly clear to me during my visit to this land. The only real differences are those of language, not of fact.

Modern man in his life's journey must make full use of whatever tools exist, drawing on all peoples and all cultures from the dawn of Creation through the latest refinements of the present. He cannot alienate himself from Truth, wherever it exists — be it in laboratories, universities, tribal cultures or in the homilies and folk sayings picked up at the knee of his own Grandma.

This is a practical book, one designed for use in everyday life. It is the first of its kind, though there will be others to follow.

I hope that it can serve to bring more joy into you own life, as it already has for many others.

Harish Johari
Oakland, California

One

The Three Gunas

Editors comment: It is interesting to note that the concept of the three Gunas, developed many thousands of years ago, is very similar to the contemporary and much publicized Bio-Rhythm which concludes that there are three rhythm patterns that control the life of every individual. You may find this chapter on The Three Gunas *heavy going. Even so, we suggest that you read it through carefully for, once you understand the interplay of inertia, activity and essences (the three Gunas) you will find the teachings of this book easier to grasp and apply to your daily life.*

Everything that exists forms one part of a vast and universal play of cosmic energy. There is nothing which has an independent existence, for any single "thing" can be shown to have direct links to other "things". Independence and individuality are in actual fact myths of human origin. Man cannot live without air. Air exists because the planetary mass of Earth and its rotational speed (and a host of other factors) enable her to cloak herself with a mantle of gases. And Earth itself exists by the grace of Sun; which in turn exists as part of the Galaxy. Galaxy exists as part of the Macrocosm.

At this point Western science stops, and enters into a realm of theoretical astrophysics and cosmogenesis. The myth of human individuality is belied by the scientific evidence, but the nature of this Universe of which man is part remains an elusive and fascinating mystery.

In India, however, man has for thousands of years seen his own role as an interdependent agent in a Macrocosmic drama. The role of man is understood as a manifestation of the same primal force which gave birth to suns and galaxies. Man is seen in the light of a complex and meaningful cosmology and ontology (science of being-as-it-is). It seems far more than coincidence that this most ancient of cosmologies is increasingly confirmed with each refinement in contemporary knowledge from the material sciences.

It is this cosmology which underlies all classical Indian science, including the science of daily life.

Most of the Indian views of Reality can be understood in Western terms. But no parallel terms exist for the forces at work at the heart of Creation, the triad which exists at the core of every phenomenon. These all-pervasive forces are the *three gunas,* called *tamas* (Inertia), *rajas* (Activity), and *sattva* (Essence).

All manifestation springs from the common source of *prakriti*. This primordial wellspring of being can be likened to an inverted tree, one whose roots are up, and trunk and branches downward. The part of the tree which is hidden from human sensory perception is the root part, the *mool-prakriti* (*mool*=root). It is this root from which all Creation arises.

Mool-prakriti, the primary existence, is the state of complete balance, or equilibrium. This *prakriti* is without gender, without identification, without form — without any qualifications to its nature. Nature here is undifferentiated, beyond all human sensory perceptions.

In this stage of undifferentiated unity, existence assumes only the purest and lightest frequencies. All at this stage is *sattva*, essence.

For this state of wholeness, *sattva* continually generates space from itself. And this generation of space is the first step in the creation cycle. For a time, space pours out freely, as water flows freely in the ocean. But once manifestation begins, the pull is inexorably downward. As the currents of space are generated, a blockage in their flow evolves as the current eddies back on itself. This blockage, this obstruction in the flow of space, is *tamas*.

It is *tamas* which is the prime cause of creation, for without obstruction *sattvic* frequencies would never begin the descent from subtle to gross.

The presence of *tamas* breaks the uniformity of the flow of space, forming an independent circuit. This new circuit, a closed system formed out of the frequencies of the root *prakriti*, is called the Golden Egg (*Hiranya Garbha* in Sanskrit).

So long as the *prakriti* is inert, motionless, nothing exists but pure *sattva*. But the generation of space creates motion, activity. It is the nature of Creation that once the play of action begins that the energy flows inevitably from high to low, from subtle to gross. Once the action starts, currents of energy are formed. And with the passage of time, it is inevitable that one current obstructs the passage of another — forming an eddy, a ripple in the stream of evolution.

By themselves, the *gunas* are imperceptible — rather, beyond perception. Only the effects of their action can be seen.

This is just as with a man. Try to *see* a man. Anything which the eye can perceive is not the *man*. The body which is seen goes through continual changes as it evolves, matures and decays. The cells are continually dying and being replaced by new growth. The tissues with which life began all die before age 12. In effect, one has a new body every 12 years. Yet there is an abiding sense of "I" which never changes, which stands beyond the changing nature of the form. It is this "I" which is the essence of a man — and this "I" is never seen.

Similarly, try to *hear* a man. What is heard is not the man, but a code of electrical signals within the listener's own brain caused by the vibration of air molecules striking the eardrum. Yet the inner sound of the man, his own rhythm cycle, exists beyond the changes of the outer sounds he makes. This sound cannot be heard by another.

So too one cannot smell another man, only the chemicals which are being given off by his body — chemicals that have their source in foods, drinks and compounds. And similarly, one cannot know the taste of another man, nor can one know his touch.

What one does experience of another is his *effect*, the gross manifestation of his being. But the real nature cannot be perceived through the senses.

Whatever is experienced of another person is just the external effect of an internal causal process happening within the other. And so too the real form of the *gunas* cannot be experienced through the senses. All that can be known is the effect of their interactions, their *maya*.

Ice, liquid and steam constitute three manifestations of the same essential substance, water. In the liquid state, the essence of water is able to flow freely within the confines dictated by the shape of its container. In ice form, this same essence has lost all mobility and has become confined to one form and one placement. In steam form, the essence is closest to its true nature, for now it fills whatever room it occupies and makes its way into all spaces, all nichés and corners.

Water is the *rajasic* form of the essence, and the transitional stage between ice and steam, and between steam and ice. To become steam, ice has first to become water; and to become ice, steam has first to become water. Ice, then, is the *tamasic* form of the essence, the form most bound by time and space, and the form in which the movement of individual particles has virtually ceased. Lastly, steam is the *sattvic* form of the essence, for steam has escaped the limits of gravity and form and dispersed into space.

If, on its journey, the subtle encounters knowledge, that knowledge immediately burns off the ignorance arising from attachment and being immediately merges with its true nature, which is pure light.

Ignorance is the path of evolution. Evolution flows in the darkness of ignorance, and in that ignorance the unlimited becomes limited, thinking itself to be a limited body.

This is the structure of the tree of *prakriti*. From the invisible roots arises a sense of individuality, the ego. The ego, in turn, creates five sense elements with which to create the world of names and forms. Next, mind arises, and with mind five sense organs and five work organs. Lastly, the physical body itself. The fruit of the tree of *prakriti* is birth, age and enjoyment, and the taste of the fruit is pleasure and pain. From pure *sattva* consciousness became active (*rajas*) and found itself pulled downward into the limitation (*tamas*) of individual form.

Consciousness has become bound by form, and while so enmeshed in its own game must obey the laws and principles governing the domain of names and forms. The three *gunas* and five elements (space, air, fire, water and earth), combined with the One consciousness, constitute the *Ashtadha Prakriti,* the eight-fold nature of manifest reality. All that exists in the world of the senses is but a play of the elements, directed by the ever-changing interaction of the *gunas* and experienced by the One consiousness.

The *gunas* can be seen as three coloured strands braided together. Sometimes one colour appears most dominant on the surface, sometimes another, sometimes another. Yet by observing the whole cord, one sees that dominance is an illusion: all three are always present, only one sometimes hides another from view. They are not three distinct entities, but three forms of one existence. The *gunas* do not disturb each other, nor do they contradict each other. Neither do they present obstacles in each other's way. One helps the other to evolve. They act together in coherence with each other, and are present in everything in varying proportions.

Scope and Power of the Gunas

Sattva is capable of producing light. It is in the light of *sattva* that one sees his dreams. The light which is seen in the dreaming state is the light of *sattva*. The eyes and all other sense organs are closed, yet darkness does not rule dreams. For this reason *sattva* is linked with the pineal hormone, Melatonin. It is *sattva* which is capable of producing light and thus removing confusion by providing a clear perspective.

Rajas has the power to activize. This *guna* motivates and inspires one to work. Its nature is pain, for pain only arises from activity.

Tamas stops. It is this *guna* which is the source of resistance, obstacles and obstructions.

Job of the Gunas

The *gunas* try to dominate each other in turn. It is very clear that one *guna* dominates at one time, while another holds sway later.

When *sattva* dominates, *rajas* and *tamas* are pushed into the background. At that time all feelings of inspiration to undertake some action vanish, as does attachment. All inspiration to work, all ignorance, vanish. There is nothing to do, nowhere to go, no job to tackle, no desire to eat, no desire to sleep, no confusion. All that remains is light and bliss — and this in turn creates more light, more peace and more tranquillity.

When *rajas* dominates it pushes *sattva* and *tamas* into the background. There is a great rush of energy, and a great desire to undertake work, projects and activity. Action is the dominant mode.

When *tamas* dominates, *rajas* and *sattva* are pushed into the wings. At this time a man feels laziness and attachment. He doesn't care to go anywhere, but would prefer to remain as he is.

The Gunas in Interaction

All three *gunas* depend on each other, and help each other in the process of evolution, and in the process of self-development as the gross evolves back towards the subtle.

In the process of bringing each other out, one *guna* serves as the stepping stone for another. A thing which is stable and *tamas*-dominated is provided motivation and activity by *rajas*, that motion and activity helps in the process of realization, as the thing moves to attain its true and essential nature — which is its light, its *sattva*. Hidden by *tamas*, *sattva* takes the help of *rajas* to bring itself into the light.

The *gunas* never become separated from each other, they always exist as one unit and one pair. When one *guna* dominates, the other two form a pair which remains recessive. But they are never completely away or absent. The *gunas* are omnipresent. *Sattva* makes a pair with *rajas*. *Tamas* makes a pair with *rajas*. Only *sattva* cannot directly join with *tamas*, for *rajas* is necessary to convert *sattva* into *tamas*, and *tamas* into *sattva*. *Tamas* has no way to approach *sattva* without *rajas*, and *sattva* has no way to approach *tamas* without help of *rajas*. Thus, *rajas* is the moderator, for without his help neither *sattva* nor *tamas* can act — for, *rajas is* activity.

Sattva then can be seen as *tamas* transformed by activity into its highest frequencies. *Tamas*, then, is *sattva* transformed by activity into its lowest frequencies.

The wax of the candle is the *tamas* of light. It needs the spark of the match on its wick (the *rajas*) to convert itself into the light (the *sattva*). The relationship between *tamas* and *sattva* is the same relationship that exists between wax and light. Was is light in its grossest form; light, the subtle form of wax.

The *gunas* are inseparable. They were neither separate ever nor can they become separate. They are only interconvertible — one can be changed into another.

Nature of the Gunas

Sattva is light — light in weight, light in its radiance and lustre and light in nature.

Rajas is activity, and its role is manifestation. When *rajas* dominates the body of a man he experiences great enthusiasm, restlessness and energy to work. It is *rajas*, by its mercurial nature, which excites *sattva* to give light.

It is *tamas* which maintains ignorance, fear and superstition. *Tamas* obscures truth behind illusion, and then makes a man fear to know it. *Tamas* is procrastination, lack of incentive and sleep. While *sattva* is purpose; *rajas* energy — *tamas* is inertia, the downward pulling force which begs one to surrender his activity.

In both *sattva* and *tamas* a man abandons the world of the senses. But in *sattva* he merges into light; while in *tamas* he merges into darkness.

These are the three cosmic forces, the *gunas*, in their nature and roles. One has seen how they operate. One knows that while *sattva* and *tamas* are exact opposites (one is light, the other darkness) they are not in fact working against each other. *Sattva* and *tamas* help each other in the process of evolution from subtle to gross, and in development from gross to subtle. They bring energy out of the lower frequencies and convert it into the higher ranges. It is not the "struggle for existence", or even the "survival of the fittest", but rather the ceaseless interplay of *gunas*.

Sattva is light, *tamas* is heavy. *Tamas* gives stability and forms the foundation stone. *Rajas* creates activity and provides inspiration.

The game of Creation is actually a play of the *gunas* and the five elements. These eight, under the witness of the One consciousness, interact to create the whole world of name and form.

Everything on the planet has pleasure, pain and attachment. There is no object which cannot give some man pleasure, some man pain and some man a sense of attachment. The sense objects either create one, two or all three responses in the individual according to his own vibrational frequencies and capacity to receive. One who is *sattva*-dominated receives pleasure. One who is *rajas*-dominated receives pain. One who is *tamas*-dominated experiences attachment. One dominated by *sattva* and *rajas* receives both pleasure and pain; one dominated by both *rajas* and *tamas* experiences pain and attachment.

Everything that exists contains within itself something with which one can identify feelings of pleasure, pain and attachment — *sattva-rajas-tamas*.

Gunas and Self-Development

The natural flow of evolution is from subtle to gross. The Universe existed first as one Cosmic Atom, or Golden Egg. Ideas exist first in the minds of men. Then comes activity, which starts a downward flow of movement. The Golden Egg shatters, the man begins to implement his idea. The downward flow of energy continues until finally energy becomes entrapped in gross form. The Solar System takes shape, the idea becomes a material product.

This play of energy can be seen in every dimension of being, for the material world of names and forms is but a product of these same forces; and the internal world of the human mind too is governed by their action.

Man is an evolute of the Universe, consciousness brought down and attached to material form.

Yet this process of evolution is not irreversible. Each man contains within himself a spark of consciousness which intuitively recalls the bliss of undifferentiated unity with the Cosmos — the very nature of consciousness. Each man has five sense organs to perceive the world, and five work organs with which to act.

From *sattva* to *rajas* to *tamas* is the natural course of evolution, yet that same *rajas* can be used to convert *tamas* back into *sattva*. With his five sense organs and five work organs man has the choice either to flow with gravity ever downward into *tamas*, or to create activity to move upwards, into light.

The *sattva*-dominated man sees a thing, and the past, present and future of that thing become clear to him. The sense object immediately is linked to the Source in his mind, and from the Source he traces its evolution through its various stages to its present form — and from the present, into the future.

The *rajas*-dominated man will see the object and fit it into his scheme of action in terms of its present value alone.

The *tamas*-dominated man will be oblivious to the object unless, perchance, he stumbles over it.

Sattva is light, clarity and understanding. *Rajas* is inspiration, activity and pain. *Tamas* is doubt, darkness and attachment.

One can choose to generate more *sattva* in his life, or to join the downward flow of energy into *tamas* (which finally ends in complete inertia, death). To increase *sattva* means to experience more pain as the *tamas* is consumed by the fire of self-discipline. But the pain gives way to light, to pleasure and to clear understanding of one's nature and role in the Universe.

One who understands the three *gunas* and their nature can recognize their presence and action within himself, and from this knowledge assume responsibility for the development of his own organism.

He will discover that some foods are *sattvic*, some *rajasic*, some *tamasic*. He will learn that his own feelings are the clearest and best guide to the workings of the *gunas* within himself — that activities and events which produce lightness, clarity and insight are *sattvic* in nature; that those things which produce inspiration, activity and pain are *rajasic;* that those things which produce attachment, doubt, ignorance and sleep are *tamasic*.

By using *rajas* to increase *sattva,* one can move counter to the natural gravitational pull and rejoin his consciousness with the One consciousness which gave him birth. The drop can merge back into the Ocean.

The prize for one who makes the effort is *sat-chit-ananda,* Truth, Being and Bliss.

Two

The Science Of Breath

The human body is an autonomous, self-synchronous organism created by consciousness for experiencing life in the world of names and forms. Included in the instrumental design are precise mechanisms for synchronizing with the rhythmic cycles of the planet and cosmos.

The most important, easily regulated and effective of these mechanisms are the two nostrils.

Each organism contains all the elements present throughout the whole of the cosmos, and all elements operate according to common rules and principles — regardless of their placement in time and space. Crystals always form along the same axis, water always freezes below 0° Centigrade. The same rules governing the play of elements in Sun, Moon, planets and stars govern the play within the human organism.

The one fundamental principle, omnipresent and eternal, is the plan of polar opposites.

A bi-polar electromagnetic field encompasses each manifested form from smallest atom to largest galaxy. In each field a positive pole expresses energy, while a negative pole draws it back into itself. The interplay between these two poles forms the phenomenal event itself, that which is called solid, liquid, fiery, gaseous — and even space itself. Without this interplay, without separation, only undifferentiated unity would exist.

The operation of each sub-field according to the same rules and principles unites all Creation into a coherent whole. As the science of cybernetics has made abundantly clear to Western man in recent years, there is no closed system but The System Itself. All events, all perceivable phenomena, are but sub-systems of the One.

The commonality of operation links all events together, and it is this principle which underlies all sciences — particularly physiology and astrology.

The Role of Breath

The nose, with its two nostrils, is the only bodily organ in continuous interplay with the external environment. The sleeping man, the unconscious man neither hears, sees, smells, tastes or touches. But he does breathe.

Through the two nostrils the human organism draws in air and vital energy, as well as all the vibrations present in the external environment in their most subtle and refined form. Breath is that which keeps man in continuous contact with the world.

The importance of breath in maintaining life cannot be discounted. What is less understood is the role of the nostrils themselves as other than conduits for the passage of air into the lungs.

If nostrils were needed solely for transporting air into the chest, surely one would have been sufficient. Man has two eyes to see in three dimensions, and two ears to be able to localize sound. But why two nostrils?

Western medical science has virtually neglected this simple yet significant question.

On careful observation one will notice that the breath does not come through both nostrils in equal volume, except for very brief periods and during cases of severe emotional disturbance. Normally, one breathes either through one or the other. Observation over time will reveal further that the breath alternates between the nostrils according to a regular pattern.

And one who makes observation of the breath a personal science will soon notice that the nature of consciousness changes according to the dominance of one nostril over the other.

The Split Brain

The answer to this enigma can be found within the confines of the skull. Here, in the form of the grey matter of the brain, electromagnetic energy in the body reaches in greatest concentration and intensity. This organ is divided into two distinct halves, the left and right hemispheres.

Only on very rare occasions is energy equally distributed in both halves of the brain. Under normal conditions, electrical activity — as manifested in the form of brainwaves — is concentrated more in one hemisphere than the other. Recent observations by brain researchers show that each hemisphere has uniquely characteristic forms of behaviour, and that these behaviours are normally present only when electrical activity centres in that hemisphere.

When energy concentrates in the left hemisphere, one becomes more active, verbal, intellectual, extroverted, creative, male and solar. Conversely, right hemisphere dominance is characterized by passivity, orientation to sight and sounds, emotional responses, introversion, femininity and lunar energy.

Only in rare moments is energy distributed equally.

At these times consciousness undergoes major changes, and one either becomes extremely tranquil or extremely agitated and disturbed.

The brain then contains the essence of the play of opposites, the eternal *Leela*.

As one's whole nature of response changes according to the movement of energy from one hemisphere to the other, each hemisphere (and the state when both operate equally) exerts a unique, readily discernible mode of operation. Perceptions, actions and even "involuntary bodily responses" vary according to the dominance of one hemisphere over the other.

Clearly, then, if a means of voluntarily controlling the localization of energy in the brain could be found, one could control his own state of consciousness at will.

Breath and the Hemispheres

The movement of energy from one hemisphere to the other occurs simultaneously with the change of breath from one nostril to the other. When right nostril dominates, left hemisphere dominates; when left nostril dominates, so does the right hemisphere. When both nostrils operate, both hemispheres operate in unison.

The simple act of changing the breath from one nostril to the other reverses brain hemisphere dominance, altering chemical reactions taking place throughout the organism. Wilful control of the pattern of breath enables conscious control of body chemistry.

Human feeling states are the product of body chemistry. Changing the breath pattern changes body chemistry, and thus affects a change in the feeling state. Disease states are the product of body chemistry. Changing the breath pattern changes body chemistry, and thus affects the prevention of disease if done at the onset of symptoms.

Knowledge and practice of the principles of breath

science enables one to control his state of consciousness and prevent disease states.

Swar Yoga

Knowledge of the play of breath in the nostrils forms the basis of the ancient discipline of *Swar Yoga* (literally, "unification through breath"), heretofore virtually unknown even in its native India.

The founders and developers of this science observed the play of breath and the resulting changes in body state and consciousness. What follows are their most significant and useful findings, information with which anyone can synchronize his own inner rhythms with those of the cosmos:

1. One does not breathe through both nostrils simultaneously except for very brief periods during the day.
2. When one nostril is dominant, the other is recessive.
3. Breath may be changed from one nostril to the other by lying down on the side of the operating nostril with a pillow placed under the ribcage (to stimulate nerves which play an important role in breath). Change, in healthy organisms. occurs within three to ten minutes.
4. When right nostril operates, body chemistry is predominantly acidic (the stomach produces more gastric acid during right nostril operation) and more inner heat is produced. This nostril should never be used for meditation, urination or drinking liquids.
5. When left nostril operates, body chemistry is predominantly alkaline. This nostril cools the system and should never be used for eating, bathing or defecating.
6. To whatever degree possible, the left nostril should be operated during the day and the right between sunset and sunrise — except when specific jobs

requiring the other nostril are undertaken. This synchronizes the organism with the type of energy most predominant on the planet. The day is more hot and solar, so the cooler nostril is used; and the reverse for nighttime.

7. When both nostrils operate equally, body chemistry reaches a state of equilibrium (stasis) suitable for no other jobs than meditation, chanting or yoga. This state occurs normally at the exact moments of sunrise and sunset and briefly during the transition from one nostril to the other (which occurs hourly in most individuals).

8. The cycle of the breath is directly related to the ascending and descending cycles of the Moon.

9. On the morning following the Darkest Night (New Moon) of the lunar cycle, left nostril begins operating at the moment of sunrise and continues for one hour. This is true also for the second and third mornings.

10. On the three consecutive mornings following the Full Moon night, right nostril begins operating at sunrise, continuing for an hour.

11. When one nostril has operated for three successive mornings, the breath will switch to the other nostril for the next three mornings, subject to variances in the 28½ day lunar cycle.

12. When there is a disturbance in the natural cycle, and the proper nostril does not open, body chemistry becomes disturbed and physiological and psychological disturbances become more likely.

13. A quick response to this imbalance can avert ill effects. Simply change the breath by the method outlined above — resorting to a cotton ball "plug" if there is no change-over. Under no circumstances should one breathe through the mouth.

14. Changing the breath at the first sign of any physical or mental disturbance prevents worsening of symptoms and promotes rapid recovery.

Mechanism of Action

The interplay of sensory stimulation, convection cooling and ionic balance links breath pattern with brain activity.

Air of a temperature at variance with normal body temperature passes through the nostrils at relatively high velocity, exciting the sensory nerves lining the inner passage. These nerves are extensions of the olfactory bulbs on the underside of either lobe — an organ directly linked to the large, complex structure of the Rhinencephalon, or "smell brain". This organ controls a vast network of associative nerves linked with every structure of the brain. And despite the fact that its primary input comes from the nerves leading to the nostrils, only a comparatively small segment of this organ deals with the sense of smell.

The intake of air also cools and dehydrates the inner surface of the nostrils and sinus cavities. Cooling slows chemical reactions in the hemisphere on the same side (right hemisphere if right nostril operates). Evaporation creates a demand for additional mucous, and additional diversion of energy from the same side hemisphere.

Electrically charged ions permeate the atmosphere and pass into the body with each inhalation — and electricity provides the mechanism of nerve action. Significantly, the breath tends to fill the lobe of the lung on the operating side more than the lobe on the non-operating side. The interaction of these two factors creates a relatively major difference in ionic stimulation of the nerve energy in the two sides of the respiratory tract and body. Right nostril breath concentrates nerve energy in the right-hand side of the body; left in the left-hand side.

Breathing through one nostril not only cools the hemisphere on the same side, but stimulates the opposite hemisphere as well. Differences in ionic stimulation, electrical activity, blood flow, and skin temperature can always be detected between the two halves of the body — except when both nostrils operate.

Breath and Lunar Cycle

Sun rules the day and is electrical and hot in nature. Moon rules the night and is magnetic and cold. Radio transmissions travel farther at night because of the lack of solar-generated electrical interference in the ionosphere and because the magnetic lunar energy is receptive by nature. This can be readily proved by anyone who listens to a distant radio station.

Right nostril is the solar nostril; left nostril is lunar. Sun and Moon form the two poles of the day cycle, and their basic natures correspond to the nature of the two hemispheres and the two nostrils.

Of the two forms of energy governing the planet, Sun is the more constant, going through an energy cycle once every 365 ¼ days — and never absent altogether during the day. Such is not the case with the Moon, however. Sometimes full and bright in the night sky, at other times not present at all; the Moon waves and wanes regularly in a 28 ½-day cycle, and governs the tides of the oceans.

Moon similarly affects the 70 per cent of human body weight which is water. Just as the tides reach their zenith on the night of the Full Moon, so too there is a high tide in the emotional lives of men. And when the tides reach their lowest ebb with the coming of the Darkest Night, human emotional power is at its weakest.

The cycle of the nostrils begins anew each fortnight with the coming of the Full or Dark Moon nights. Lunar power crests on Full Moon night and begins its descent. At this time solar power is increasing, and so the right nostril will operate for the hour following the coming of dawn. Similarly, solar power peaks on the Darkest Night and Lunar energies begin to build anew — and so left nostril will operate after sunrise.

Sleep-Fasts

These two celestial events mark the extremes of energy present on the planet. And by remaining awake on these two nights (not sleeping until the following evening after the sun has set), one can sensitize his system even more acutely to the natural rhythms of the planet.

Swar Yoga texts stress the extreme significance of sleep-fasting on these two nights. Regular practice of this discipline synchronizes the cycle of the nostrils and helps free the system from dullness, drowsiness and inertia.

Nostrils, Jobs and Healing

Each breath — right nostril, left nostril and joint operation of the two — creates specific psychophysiological ·states. A task undertaken during the operation of one nostril may or may not be suited for that state of body chemistry. Left nostril is more suitable for all long-term peaceful activities not undertaken for immediate gain. Right nostril is best suited for all unstable, short-term jobs undertaken for immediate gain; as well as hard physical labour. Joint operation is appropriate only for concentration, meditation, worship and chanting.

Left Nostril Jobs: building a house, starting any new business, charity, dancing, curing depression, talking to one's elders or superiors, drinking non-alcoholic beverages, meeting or talking with friends and loved ones, gardening, entering a new house, getting married, playing music, meditating, depositing money, entering a holy order, buying and wearing jewellery, curing pain, reading or writing poetry, learning to read, curing sorrow and unconsciousness, making short journeys, practising yoga, and entering a new phase in one's educational career.

Right Nostril Jobs: attracting others, bathing, boat trips, reading or writing books, courtship, debating, defecating, eating, enjoying, gambling, gem cutting, giving inspiration to others, hard physical labour, removing anxiety and nervousness, learning musical compositions, sleeping, mastering religious texts, long journeys, warfare, woodcutting and *hatha yoga* exercises.

Additionally, males should use the right nostril during sexual contact; females, the left.

Three

The Glory Of Waking Up

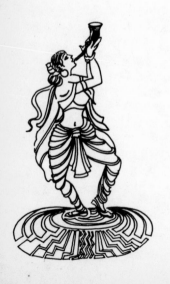

The pulse of the cosmos mirrors itself in the human body, with the beating of the heart reflecting the throbbing rhythm of the universe itself. The same elements which comprise the mantle of this earth are the very elements making up the human body, and the laws which govern their form and actions are the same, "as within, so without".

We, each one of us, comprise a microcosmic manifestation of all the elements, all the laws existing throughout Creation. To separate man from his place as an evolute of the cosmos is to deny the very core of Reality.

We cannot escape. We are all products of the same omnipresent, omnipotent and omniscient Causal Principle.

But we can hide, we can deny. We can veil ourselves in the illusion of "free will" and "self-determinism". Nonetheless each of us somehow has two eyes, two ears, two nostrils, two arms, two legs and one mouth and one anus. Each must breathe. Each must eat. Each must sleep.

Physics tells us that when two or more vectors of force

interact, a new flow is created following the path of least resistance. Man is a product of the vectors of cosmic force, and has within himself an inborn flow, an innate direction. By denying the principles which gave him birth, man can resist or divert the flow. But the price is pain and a sense of separation, anxiety and loneliness.

Yoga is the science of seeking out the flow which rises and falls in each of us; then tuning in and harmonizing one's existence with this flow.

Dharma is the flow, and *karma* the means by which one can re-establish contact with this all-pervading Essence. The first stage is the realization that one is an evolute of the cosmos. Only then can one begin to bring his own discordant rhythms into harmony with the larger patterns of the cosmic symphony.

The same sun rises and sets each day for all beings. And throughout the world the daily cycle of light and dark establishes the basic cycle for all life forms.

With the first stirring of dawn, about 90 minutes before the sun appears over the eastern horizon, comes a great surge of energy on the planet.

Sleeping creatures awaken, shaking the vestiges of inertia from their systems in preparation for the activities of the day.

Then, less than a half hour before sunrise, a second surge of energy rushes through the atmosphere, this one still more powerful. With this second indraft of radiation comes the single most important moment of the day — the time when body chemistry is set for all living beings.

Man is also affected by this cycle. Physiologists from Japan found a sudden and dramatic shift in the blood chemistry of human subjects inevitably occuring within 10 or 20 minutes of the sun's appearance.

The blood at this time is thinned and suffused with fresh chemicals, which gradually exhaust themselves — only to be restored again at the next sunrise.

Physical health and emotional well-being are both the products of body chemistry, a fact demonstrated by the changes in both states produced by the addition of foreign chemicals (drugs) to the system. If drugs can produce changes in physical and emotional states, both must themselves be reflections of body chemistry.

This brings us to the First and most important step in harmonizing individual being — rising at least 45 minutes before dawn.

The suffusion of the system with new energy takes place ten minutes before sunrise, whether or not we are consciously prepared and awake — but how much better if we are prepared.

Chemical reactions take place best in clean vessels, free from contaminants. Our own bodies are vessels of chemical reactions. Logic dictates that a reaction taking place in a vessel free from wastes and contaminants will produce much greater results than a reaction in an impure vessel.

During sleep the human system centralizes all wastes and refuse products in the bowels and bladder. The lower abdomen is full of waste-charged gases which will be used on awakening to push the urine and stool out of the system.

If one is sleeping at sunrise, these gases and wastes will be present during the setting of blood chemistry. If one is awake, bowels and bladder emptied, body cleansed, and sitting in a receptive mood at sunrise, how much different would be the outcome?

Throughout history, all religions in all parts of the world have stressed to one degree or another the importance of rising before dawn and greeting the new day refreshed and receptive. The Hindu tradition lists failure to meditate in these early morning hours as one of the Fourteen Failings.

Only a healthy person can enjoy living in this world, and the first key to bodily health is rising 10 minutes or more before dawn. Sanskrit scriptures call this time

Brahma Mahoorta or *Amrit Bela*. *Brahma Mahoorta* means the *"time of Brahma"*, pure consciousness, the Divine Self. *Amrit Bela* signifies the time of the nectar of life.

During these crucial minutes the body's glaze of health increases, as do physical strength and the powers of concentration. One is filled with fresh energies, inspired to undertake any kind of work — and any project initiated at this time is always completed. Difficult problems requiring great mental effort are most easily solved, and memory is at its sharpest. Sick persons feel released from the agonies which kept them awake and troubled through the night, often falling into deep, replenishing sleep.

Only in the past 50-60 years have people in civilized nations neglected rising before dawn. And it is these same 50-60 years which have heralded an unprecedented upsurge in heart disease, cancer and a score of other disorders — as well as the birth and phenomenal growth of the psychiatric and psychological professions.

Morning Practices

Modern man has once again to understand the importance of early morning rising. He has forgotten those practices which should be followed after waking to tune in body and mind. Each morning is the start of a new day. "Today is the first day of the rest of your life."

What purpose in a new day if we allow ourselves to get entangled in the trips of the previous day? By allowing our energies to be spent in pondering the previous day's follies and fortunes, the advantages gained by rising before dawn are exhausted in a destructive fashion. Receiving energy is important, but equally critical is the manner in which we spend it.

Of first importance is never to take any food or drink in the pre-dawn hours. Many people are addicted to a cup of coffee or tea, even before setting foot out of bed. In India, where tea is the national beverage, this practice is prevalent among Western-oriented people and is called "bed tea" by the traditional majority. It must be considered a crime against the system. For what one is doing is adding a chemical stimulant to the system before emptying the bowels and bladder.

Morning is a time to keep one's speed slow and easy. Adding a stimulant not only speeds up the system, but causes the waste-charged gases to move upward, circulating throughout the body.

Tuning In

On gaining consciousness one should place his hand slightly below his nose to see which of his two nostrils is open. Once you have discovered which nostril is working, you should work with that side of the body first, for that's where the energies are more concentrated. Centre your attention where your energy is already centred and you will be in harmony with your own natural cycles.

If you are breathing through your right nostril, look at the palm of your right hand. Observe the lines and patterns. Study it closely, recognize it as your best friend, then kiss it. The act of kissing confers energy — and by kissing your palm, you give your best vibrations to your most effective tool for self-expression.

Now observe your palm branching out, spreading out to become five channels of energies ending in your fingertips. Through the palm and its five extensions have come virtually all of mankind's highest expression. Poetry, painting, sculpture, music, architecture and countless art forms have taken birth from the human mind through this palm and fingers. Know then that you are contemplating your greatest implement for good or evil in the world. Unimaginable power flows through the fingers. With one gesture of one extended finger a single man can influence a multitude.

This power is reflected in the extraordinary proportion of the brain devoted to the hands, far exceeding most other parts of the body. Smokers know they consume more cigarettes when nervous, and that their anxiety is allayed in large part by the simple act of manipulating the cigarette with their fingertips. This same principle of engaging conscious energy through the fingertips operates in the use of rosaries and prayer wheels.

Concentration of energy in the hands will divert attention from straying thoughts and centre awareness in the present. After looking at your palm, kissing it and looking at your fingers, rub their tips together with the thumbs in a slow, soothing rhythm cycle.

Of all parts of the body the hands and face convey the greatest range of expressions. We learn to mask our emotions with our faces by donning social masks, but to the astute observer our hands inevitably betray our real emotional state. In anger, the clenched fist and white knuckles reveal the rage within. In anxiety, we may "grasp at straws" and pick at lint or our fingernails. Wrapped in enthusiasm we gesture spontaneously and effusively. In repression, we literally "hold ourselves in." And the artist, lost in his work, moves fluidly, almost poetically.

When sitting or standing our spine is at a 90-degree angle to the earth, and gravity automatically pulls energy down into the hands. So when we awaken in the morning, this simple routine ensures a proper flow of energy into the hands and helps bring their actions under conscious control.

Following the exercise of the fingertips, one should twist his wrist in a clockwise direction to loosen up the muscles and give free motion. Then inhale a few deep breaths of the fresh morning air and sit silently with an empty mind for a few seconds, avoiding any interaction with others. Avoiding conversation helps maintain the gentle early morning vibration and protects one from negative thoughts.

Getting Out of Bed

With your system now calm and relaxed, step out of bed with the same foot as the operating nostril. This sequence of motions, starting with observing and kissing your palm, forms an energy shield which wards off negative influences for the whole of the day.

"I got out of bed on the wrong side." How many times have you unthinkingly uttered these words without understanding that a great truth is hidden in them?

We have already mentioned that the nostrils are governed by a natural cycle. Observing their operation, observing your own system, particularly your hand, and then stepping out of bed with the foot on the same side as the operating nostril brings you into harmony with the energies present on the planet.

Surely you have noticed that on mornings when you have awakened late and been forced to leap out of bed, everything seems jumbled and chaotic. Simply by performing these few simple waking-up rituals, you can avert all disorder by starting the day in a slow-paced, orderly fashion, as the start of any undertaking plays a crucial role in determining the outcome.

Once out of bed, sit down for a minute or two before a mirror and smile at yourself, make a few faces and enjoy your image. By this simple act you free your facial muscles of tensions and avoid the worst of all morning ailments, seriousness. So be expressive, let your clown out. Then see how hard it is to be serious about yourself. Children perform this exercise spontaneously.

Hindu scriptures also proclaim the benefits of seeing something white at this time, especially yogurt, white flowers or white birds. A cow or a deer is also good. All these are soothing visuals which calm and relax the system. None is likely to produce a chain of negative thoughts.

Under no circumstances should you see anyone with a long face or a person who is angry. All these sights, a long face, a miser, a sinner, a criminal, or a person who is angry. All these sights drain energy and are likely to cause disturbing thought patterns throughout the course of the day, just as diverting a river at the source alters its whole course to the sea. If one of these visuals is present, close your eyes until it is gone, or look immediately in another direction and move out of the room.

And whatever you do, don't speak to anyone. Try to keep your mind clear of thoughts. Seeing only right visuals and performing conscious tuning-in actions keeps you free from bad vibrations, and conversation can easily throw you back into them.

It is a good idea to take a slow walk in the fresh morning air, breathing deeply and slowly of the atmosphere which is charged with vital energy. Don't walk fast. Conserve your energies. This morning walk fills the system with *prana*, vital energy, and stimulates the downward flow of gases necessary for a clear bowel movement.

Cleansing the Lower Tract

First of all, it is a very bad habit to jump out of bed and run to the bathroom. You should never set foot out of bed without first checking the nostrils and performing the tuning-in exercises. After performing these activities and taking a brief stroll in the fresh air, check your nostrils again. If the right is working, defecate; if left, urinate, then change to right to defecate.

Under no circumstances should one spend too much time on the toilet as it can disturb the gases of the lower tract, resulting in a whole host of ailments, major and minor. Many people read while sitting on the toilet waiting for the bowels to move. This is a potentially dangerous habit. Newspapers are especially bad, because they often blow negative events out of proportion. And the news is already a day old by the time it appears in print, so what you are doing is locking yourself into yesterday's negative vibrations. But reading of any kind is bad at this time for two important reasons: first, energy is needed in the bowels, and reading brings it to the head; second, reading encourages sitting for prolonged periods in a posture which can cause many ailments. Keep reading matter in your study, not the bathroom.

Most bowel complaints can be eliminated if only one adopts the proper posture in defecation. The invention of the modern toilet seat ushered in an era of tremendous human suffering from constipation to allied bowel disorders. One is forced to sit in an unnatural position which demands that force be applied in a very dangerous fashion. Hemorrhoids and many other anal constrictions can be linked directly to the appearance of the toilet seat.

Good health practice dictates that defecation be done in the only natural position, the one you have been forced to use when out camping or walking. Crouch or squat. This is the posture which man has always used, except in modern "civilized" society and will quickly reduce and then eliminate hemorrhoids. This stance opens the anus fully without the need of applying force. In most Asian and many European nations even flush toilets have small platforms at either side of the bowl to allow easy adoption of this stance. But Americans will just have to balance on the outer rims of the bowl, (seat down — bare feet up when wearing shoes) which works well enough, especially if there is a nearby wall which can be used as support.

Once the bowels have moved, the anus should be cleaned with cold water. Surprisingly, toilet paper is a very poor means of cleansing and can actually irritate the sensitive tissues. Water, however, can never irritate and is an electrical conductor as well.

Water draws electrical energy to the surface of the body, vitalizing the system and insuring the proper distribution of energy throughout the organism. It prevents skin dryness as well.

All the nerves of the digestive tract, a continuous passage from mouth to anus, connect at the plexus in the anal spinctre. In defecation pressure is brought to bear on all these nerves by the muscular contractions which expel the stool. By washing with cold water, electrical energy is drawn to the surface. This action stimulates the entire nervous system, including the brain.

Importance of Bowel Movements

Why all this emphasis on regular bowel movements? The importance of clean, regular movements immediately following performance of the waking up rituals cannot be stressed too heavily. Good health depends on the proper flow of gases in the system, which in turn is dependent on the proper discharge of bodily wastes.

Because no meditation, no concentration and no physical activities, and no eating or drinking should be done before defecation, chronic morning constipation is the greatest single enemy of *sadhana* (spiritual discipline).

Preliminary Cleansing

Following urination and defecation one should always thoroughly wash the hands and face. In the morning one should clean the teeth and eyes as well.

The skin temperature rises during sleep. Blankets keep the skin temperature considerably above room temperature, especially in a room where windows have been left open to insure adequate circulation of fresh air.

Washing helps bring the system into proper equilibrium with the conditions in the room and prevents the kind of shock brought on by the sudden change in temperature of immediately leaping into a hot or cold shower.

The face, especially the eyes, should be washed with

refreshing cool water, just slightly below room temperature.

It should be remembered that the whole face is one unit, and should be treated as such in cleaning. Partial cleaning can create problems because of the difference in temperature and electrical conductivity between the cleaned and uncleaned parts. These differences can cause an imbalance in energy, affecting vision, sinuses, hearing and taste.

The eyes represent the element of fire in the body. They work only when stimulated by light. Water is the fuel of fire. What remains after fire is only dry ash because the water has been burned off. Water conducts the heat and electrical energy of the fire. So by splashing water in the eyes, the small amount of force applied by the hands electrically charges the water — stimulating and soothing the eyes and the optic nerves (which are direct extensions of the brain).

When cleaning the eyes, first fill the mouth with water, then splash water of the same temperature into the eyes. Indian texts prescribe splashing the eyes several times while swishing water through the teeth.

The eyes can also be cleaned with a few drops of rosewater (which should be refrigerated in a blue bottle when not in use). Honey and mustard oil are also excellent cleansers. As these latter two create a burning sensation, you may want to use them only at night when the eyes do not have to be opened again. For more advice on improving the sight, see the section on Ayurvedic remedies.

Just remember this little saying:

"Whenever you wash your hands, wash your face. Whenever you wash your mouth, wash your eyes."

Cleaning the ears and nose is also a good daily practice. Only mustard oil or hydrogen peroxide should be used for the ears, because the dirt which collects there is not water soluble. Just put a few drops of either liquid in the ears; allow to soak for a minute or two, then remove with a cotton swab.

Cleaning the nose should be understood as cleaning the forehead from the inside. We inhale a lot of chemicals, which we perceive as smells. These chemicals become lodged in the nose and sinus cavities. So cleaning the nose accomplishes many functions and should be included as part of routine cleansing. The best method is to suck some lukewarm water through the nostrils, spitting it out through the mouth. This may feel strange — even discomforting — the first time, but this feeling vanishes after it has been done once. This method works best with a pint of lukewarm water to which a tea-spoon each of salt and butter have been added.

After washing, apply a few drops of mustard, sesame, olive or mineral oil in each nostril, letting it stand for a minute, then rinsing again.

Brushing the teeth is always important. Indians use a fresh twig which they chew on one end to break it down into fibers which can penetrate the gaps between the teeth. A toothbrush will suffice. Use with toothpaste, powder or baking soda. Dental floss may be used as well.

Modern devices using pressurized water may also be used, but not more than weekly because the vibrations of the electrical pumps can be disturbing in the early morning hours. Whatever you do, just remember to rinse the eyes along with the mouth.

Natural Functions

For creating and maintaining physical and mental well-being, one rule stands forth above all others: *never suppress natural functions of the organism*. The vast majority of man's diseases stem from violations of this rule. "Don't go to the bathroom during class — wait 'til afterwards." "Be a man, hold it." "That's not polite." From commandments like these stem a host of physiological and mental disturbances.

The only path to good health is the observance of one's own being, paying heed to all the calls of nature. What happens when we ignore these bodily cues? Following is a partial list of answers:

Suppression of URINATION causes: bladder pain, aching genitals, inability to urinate, headache, distension of abdominal muscles, diseases of the genito-urinary system and mental confusion.

Withholding DEFECATION: intestinal cholic, constipation, retention of feces and flatus, cramps in the cal-muscles, abdominal distension, confusion, anxiety, dullness, drowsiness, anger, fatigue, pain in the abdominal region and a host of other disorders.

Stopping the urge to VOMIT: pruritis, wheals, anorexia, anemia, fever, dermatosis, nausea and acute spreading infection.

Forcing back a SNEEZE: neck stiffness, headache, facial paralysis, facial twitch, loss of sensory perceptions and migraine headache.

Suppressing BELCHING: hiccough, dyspepsia, anorexia (loss of appetite), tremor, heart and lung disorders.

Restraining YAWNING: chronic muscular spasticity, spasms, contractions, numbness, tremor and shaking.

Ignoring pangs of HUNGER: emaciation, weakness, discoloration, body ache, anorexia and giddiness.

Failure to quench THIRST: parching of throat and mouth, fatigue, depression, cardiac pain and deafness.

Holding back TEARS: chronic inflammation of nasal passages, eye disease, cardiac disorders, anorexia and giddiness.

Forgoing SLEEP: yawning, body ache, torpor, diseases of the head and heaviness of the eyes.

Not maintaining DEEP BREATHING: cardiac disorders, stupefaction, chronic tension of chest and abdominal muscles, tension, anxiety and countless other disorders.

The Role of Flowers

Contact with flowers in the earliest hours of the day refreshes and energizes the human system in a most pleasing and beneficial manner. Not only are flowers visually attractive, but they have a psychic link with the human mind. The flower is the most evolved part of the plant, the *essence* of the plant. It is the flower for which the whole plant sprouts, grows and develops. The flower is the part which reproduces the whole plant in its microcosmic seed form.

Flowers are the *sattvic* part of the plants, and contact with them during the pre-dawn and early morning hours charges the human system with *sattvic* energy.

Flowers can be divided into two broad categories on the basis of colour and smell. The first group is flowers which have strong colours but little or no smell. The second group consists of the relatively colourless flowers which nonetheless have a strong fragrance. The purpose of both colour and odour is to attract insects for pollination, the most *sattvic* of purposes — for it is this pollination which keeps the link of consciousness growing.

The colour of the flower reflects the colour of the season, and by seeing these natural seasonal hues the human nervous system is attuned to the energy of the moment. The same is true for the fragrance of the pollen, which is a factor to attune the human nervous system to the energy of the moment by stimulating the olfactory system.

The pollen also contains complex combinations of chemicals which provide the system with highly concentrated *sattvic* energy in a form directly assimilable by the tissues.

It is customary to use flowers as an offering to God. The flower, because of its fragrance, symbolizes the purest form of the earth element. The human body is made of earth — the skin, flesh, bones, hair, nerves and capillaries all are earth.

The freshness and delicacy of flowers also serves as a psychic link between man and plant. Literature is full of the praises of flowers, and poets compare endlessly the glories of flowers with human fantasies. Flowers also have a tremendous effect on human sexuality and increase stamina and pleasure in both sexes.

Similarly, there are hundreds of diseases cured by wearing flowers. One who wears bouquets or garlands finds the glamour and glaze of his complexion enhanced, evil influences dissipated, sexual energy increased and disease banished and wealth increases. For these reasons alone flowers should be made a part of everyday life.

Colourful flowers also help the human organism by absorbing the outgoing current of energy radiated by the body and giving their own coloration back into the system. Flowers also pick up human emotional vibrations. They stay alive longer if properly cared for and attended.

Fragrant flowers have a more magical effect and are more sensitive to human vibrations; their colour is generally very light and more visually soothing than the brighter flowers, and thus are more pleasant and beneficial.

Of all flowers, the lotus is most beneficial. Of those commonly available in the United States, the wild rose is best. Not only does it provide pleasing smells and visuals, but its leaves are edible and, when mixed with sugar and cardamom and kept in direct sunlight in a sealed glass jar for 40 days, provide a good tonic which soothes body chemistry and is nourishing to the heart. The sight and smell of roses alone are tonic for troubled hearts and those who have suffered serious heart ailments. Rosewater used in food also soothes the heart, and it is a good cleanser for the eyes and prevents many eye disorders.

Four

Energizing Your Body Through Massage

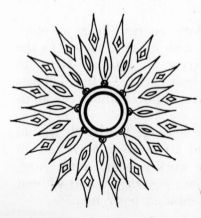

Few daily practices offer as much pleasurable benefit — or as much potential harm — as does the morning massage. Done according to the natural laws of human anatomy and energy flow, regular massage vibrates and energizes skin, muscles and nerves simultaneously.

Body heat and vitality increase as the heart and circulatory system open up to provide fresh oxygen and vital energy to all parts of the system — while simultaneously flushing out waste gases and chemicals.

Yet few practices are as potentially harmful as massage contrary to the principles on which the human body has been constructed. Any practice which creates feelings of pain automatically raises the level of tension and resistance in the organism, paving the way for structural imbalances. Permanent damage can result from improper massage techniques.

Properly executed however, massage helps the body to become light, active and energetic. Massaging regularly, even once weekly, prevents development of most skin disorders — including eczema, blisters, scabies and seborrhea. So too massage increases intelligence, ready wit, stamina, sexual vitality (semen), self-confidence and beauty.

Why Oil Massage?

Of all massage practices, those involving the use of oils are of greatest benefit. The body should never be massaged when dry, for friction, heat and pain are then produced which cause harm to the organism and disturb the balance of gases in the body. Oil softens the skin, lubricates against friction, disperses heat evenly and provides glaze, strength and resistance to extremes of temperature in the environment — as well as sudden changes in pressure.

Oils prevent dryness, increase suppleness and durability, preventing many of the effects of premature aging.

Indians routinely place oil in anus, genitals, nose, eyes, ears and navel as both a cleansing and lubricating process — just as any machine user regularly oils equipment to prevent the friction which can quickly ruin costly parts.

Oil is pure fire, pure caloric energy. Place a cotton wick in a saucer full of oil and strike a match to the wick and the oil burns, leaving no residue. Here, in liquid form, is concentrated heat energy — fire. Oil eats friction because it conducts heat readily without evaporating.

For the smoothest possible massage the hands should be lightly coated with oil, and a few drops sprinkled on that part of the body where work is being done. Now, smooth, regular movements are possible — and without the pain of dry friction or abraded body hair.

Principles of Massage

One who follows the natural contours and flows of the body insures the most effective possible massage. One who works counter to these creates imbalance and disease.

To understand the body, one need but look at the formation and function of musculature. To this end the organism can be divided into three general regions: first the torso and head — the region from the base of the spine to the top of the head; second, the region from the pelvis to the toes; third, from collarbones to fingertips.

The shape of muscles in the first division — from skullcap to tailbone — is round, and the energy flows from up to down and from down to up. In the second sector, energy moves down from pelvis to feet as the body pushes against the Earth and force of gravity with the legs. This is the part of the body designed for the function of pushing. In the third section, the upper arm, elbow, forearm, wrist, palm and fingers form a coordinated whole to draw energy into the body. This is the pulling section. In both the second and third regions, the formation of musculature is linear, and energy flows from the torso downwards or outwards.

Though the hands are used to draw energy into the body, the fingertips discharge a great deal of energy. There are many miracles related to the sensation of touching, and the transference of energy through the fingertips from one man to another (or from God to man, as Michelangelo depicted on the ceiling of the Sistine Chapel). And fingertips always point the way.

According to the structuring of each of these three major divisions, the oil must be applied accordingly. When working on front part of the torso, the hands should move downwards from face to neck to chest to abdomen to waist. On the backside, however, the hands should move upwards from the base of the spine to the top of the skull, and outwards in the area of the ribcage.

Massage of the second region begins from the region of the navel in the front, and the junction of spine and pelvis in the back — and moves down on both sides to the toes. Similarly, massage of the third region begins at the collarbones and works outward and downward to the fingertips.

If massage of the back portion of the torso is begun at the neck and moved downward along the spine to the pelvis, energy is drawn down with the hands. Most sexual games begin in this manner, with petting of the rear of the skull and the hands gradually moving downward. This flow of energy works counter to the principles of massage and should not be used except for sex play.

Application of oil at the juncture of spine and skull calms the whole nervous system, strengthens memory and improves eyesight. Application at the top of the cranium near the temples, followed by massage of the whole head, is similarly very beneficial for memory, eyesight, hearing, and hair and scalp health. Oil may be applied in the region of heart and navel, armpit, pubic area, and soles and calves of feet. Particular attention to these crucial energy centres vitalizes the whole body.

Which Oils to Use?

There are several oils which may be used in massage:

MUSTARD OIL: Organic oils are best in all cases, for whatever one applies to the skin is in some part absorbed into the body through the pores. Mustard oil is extremely beneficial because it has the power to cleanse the pores. This is the only oil which may be applied in the eyes without causing harm, and no other oils should be used in nose, ears, throat or anus and genitals. Mustard oil also has a great power to strengthen the skin and enhance pigmentation.

OLIVE OIL: Another organic oil with many good attributes. It is particularly useful for those living in cold climates, for it makes the body healthy and more receptive to solar radiation.

SESAME OIL: A good massage oil, and used as the base in making special preparations for massage. One should be certain to purchase the oil of *black* sesame seeds only. White sesame seed oil causes premature grayness when applied on the hair, while the black seed oil absorbs more *prana* (vital energy).

NATURAL OIL, MINERAL OIL: While acceptable, these are poor substitutes for the plant-based oils.

BABY OIL: These are generally non-organic, and invariably have an aroma which is unnatural. Mineral oil is preferable.

Oil Formulas

Here are some oil mixtures designed specifically for special tasks:

1. *General body massage:* To one quart mustard oil add one ounce of oil (not essence) of sandalwood. If there is a dry skin condition, add three tablespoons of wheat germ oil. For a man's massage, add a pinch of turmeric to increase virility. Heat the turmeric in a small portion of the mustard oil until it dissolves. Filter, strain and then add to the mixture.

2. *Head massage:* Mix one pint mustard oil with one ounce sandalwood oil and two ounces of almond oil. This blend is excellent for memory, wits and intelligence.

3. *For areas afflicted with numbness, cold and poor circulation:* Mix one dram each of wintergreen and eucalyptus oils with one ounce olive oil and a quart of mustard oil. This mixture provides heat and stimulates the flow of energy.

4. *Chest cold massage:* Heat one quart mustard oil on

medium-high burner, adding two garlic cloves when the oil is hot. Allow the garlic to completely char. Let cool, then massage onto chest region with a pinch of salt. This mixture should be stored for later use in a red bottle.

5. *Young women:* Instead of the heat-producing mustard oil mixture, young women should massage with an oil made of one quart of black sesame seed oil blended with an ounce of sandalwood oil.

6. *Women over 40:* Use the same basic blend from number 5, adding an ounce of almond oil to give protein to the skin.

7. *Women over 50:* Mix one-half quart black sesame oil with an equal amount of coconut oil, adding an ounce each of sandalwood, wheat germ and almond oils.

8. *Newlyweds and young people:* To one quart coconut oil add one pint of organic jasmine oil, an ounce of almond oil and a half-ounce of wheat germ oil.

9. *For excess body heat:* Black sesame oil and essence of rose oil.

10. *For women's hair:* Bhringraj oil (imported from India) strengthens, lengthens and improves colour tone.

As oils have the ability to absorb and store the effects of light frequencies when stored in bottles of different colours, mixtures may be stored in tinted bottles in direct sunlight for 40 days to produce special effects. This practice is described in greater detail in the LIGHT AND MEDICINE section of the Home Remedies chapter.

Briefly, an oil kept in a red bottle becomes hotter in nature while the same oil stored in a blue bottle becomes cooler. Where extra heat is required, keep mixtures one, three and four in a red bottle (or make from oil which has been kept in a red bottle). The cooling effect of blue light suits itself to mixtures two and nine.

One should make a practice especially of keeping blue

bottle mustard oil around the house, for oil (kept refrigerated) is the best first aid treatment for burns. Hail water, kept frozen, is also a good burn remedy.

Head Massage

Oil applied to the head is absorbed into the roots of the hair, which are in turn connected with nerve fibres leading directly to the brain. Oil strengthens the hair and reduces dryness — which is responsible for brittle hair and many scalp disorders. Third, by relaxing muscles and nerves, fatigue is eliminated from the system.

Massage of the forehead also calms the system and creates good feelings in the brain, making one feel light and "high".

Massage of the temples improves eyesight and creates a centred state of awareness.

Massage of the eyebrows relaxes the whole body, and is especially beneficial for the eyes.

Massage of the forehead increases the powers of vision and concentration.

And massage in general increases circulation and promotes relaxation. Head massage in particular increases the supply of fresh oxygen in the brain, as well as the level of pranic energy. And scalp massage can help prevent loss of hair.

Head massage should be included in the daily schedule.

WHAT OIL TO USE: For head massage, males should use if possible a 1:32 mixture of sandalwood oil and mustard oil (one-half ounce sandalwood oil — *non essence* — to one pint of mustard oil). Olive oil or black sesame oil may also be used. Women will get best results for their hair and scalp from coconut oil; and jasmine oil (again, *not essence*) is also very beneficial.

Foot Massage

A simple mustard oil massage of the feet nightly, before retiring, cures numbing of the feet, prevents cold-weather cracking and peeling of skin, reduces or eliminates infections caused by fungi and bacteria, reduces agitation and promotes sound sleep.

According to ancient Indian *Shastras* (scriptures), "Diseases do not go near one who massages his feet before sleep, just as snakes do not approach the eagles."

Simply follow the natural contours of the foot.

The Cleansing Massage

Indian folk healers have evolved a practice which combines the best elements of cleansing the body with all the benefits of daily massage. This is the process known as *ubtan*.

Once begins by making a paste of one cup of garbanzo (chickpea) or whole wheat flour, one-half cup mustard oil, and a teaspoon of turmeric. After thoroughly blending, add enough water to make a paste the consistency of light cake batter. The paste of *ubtan* should be applied over the whole body, including the hair. When the mixture begins to dry and crack, it should be removed by rubbing — following the same principles of movement outlined earlier.

According to Indian folk medicine, application of *ubtan* cures disorders caused by imbalance of mucous, increases semen, enhances strength and stamina, stimulates circulation and cures diseases and infections of the skin. Use of *ubtan* on the face relaxes the jaw and cheek muscles, and provides a healthy and clear complexion.

As soap is the greatest enemy of the skin by stripping the much-needed natural oils and chemicals and dessicating the pores, so *ubtan* is the greatest cleanser and friend. The turmeric added to the mixture provides iodine in a form which can be directly absorbed through the skin, stimulating the nerves throughout the system. The oil and flour both cleanse and lubricate — and the oil creates smoothness and glow.

The initial application of the paste draws excess heat out of the system, due in large part to the presence of iodine in the turmeric. The rubbing which begins after the paste begins to dry restores normal temperature, and draws fresh energy to the surface of the entire organism.

As discussed in the chapter on semen, semen is carried by the bloodstream throughout the body — drawn into and expelled by the prostate and testicles only as triggered by the pituitary gland in the brain. According to Indian folk medicine, this *Bindu* (as semen is known) is responsible for the glowing shine (*Ojas*) which appears on the faces of young children and healthy adults. By applying *ubtan* the semen is strengthened and diseases of skin and all three elements of body chemistry are cured in the due course of time.

(Note: If one prefers a separate oil massage, a mixture of dry oil and turmeric may be used to remove the excess oil from the skin, in the same proportions as used in the paste. This approximates the effects of the *ubtan* paste.)

Who Should Not Massage?

One who is suffering from fever should not be massaged, nor should anyone who is constipated or troubled by vomiting. Those who have taken purgatives or the *basti* practice of *Kriya Yoga* should also avoid massage.

Massage and Lymph

Massage works directly with the three circulatory systems of human body: blood, nervous and lymphatic. The lymphatic system is most directly benefited by proper massage, and most easily damaged by improper techniques.

To understand the importance of lymph in massage, it is necessary to understand the functions of this complex system of nodes, ducts and passages. The lymphatic system restores protein lost from blood capillaries to the intercellular spaces and transfers absorbed fats and fluids from the intestines to the blood circulatory system.

The lymphatic system also assists blood circulation by draining excess liquid from the bloodstream and easing the heart's workload. It is the lymphatic system also which provides a direct line of defence for the body through its army of lymphocytes, phagocytes and antibody-producing tissues.

This complex and essential system can be stimulated into more healthy functioning through exercise, compression of the individual nodes (or pressure points, as they are called), by the application of heat (fomentation) and by respiration (deep breathing practices).

By stimulating lymph flow and generating heat through friction and through the application of oils, massage cleanses and vitalizes the body without causing the buildup of toxins and ennervation which frequently accompany exercise. For this reason alone, massage is ideal for older persons whose bodies can no longer readily replenish the vital fluids lost in strenuous exercise, nor stand the strain on age-weakened muscles and tendons.

Increased lymph flow reduces blood pressure, while the relief from aches and tensions promotes a deeper, more natural breathing pattern.

Regular massage relaxes the system and aids digestion by maintaining a proper balance and circulation of body gases and fluids.

Five

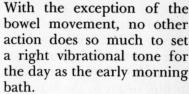

Bathing :
A Way
To Vitality

With the exception of the bowel movement, no other action does so much to set a right vibrational tone for the day as the early morning bath.

Daily bathing purifies mind and body, increases semen, promotes longevity, relieves fatigue, stops perspiration, increases strength, provides the vital glow of health, removes sleep, allays irritation, removes itch, and slakes chronic thirst.

The virtues of the bath are beyond enumeration. Good for all work organs and sense organs, the bath purifies the nerves, cures dullness and drowsiness, dissolves sorrow, creates elation, increases enthusiasm and gives vital energy to the system. So much from one simply daily routine!

As with all practices, bathing can create as many problems as it solves if approached in the wrong manner. Bathing more than twice daily should be avoided as it overtaxes the system. Similarly, baths in either very hot or very cold water should be avoided.

Cold water baths increase the amount of cold in the

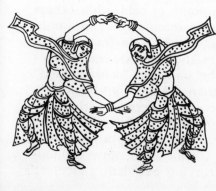

system; heat expands the muscles, gradually making them loose and flaccid. Cold water increases cold in the nerves and can lead to many varieties of muscular pain. The effects of either practice may not be experienced in youth — but if continued, will certainly manifest later in life, often in the form of weakness, cramping, kidney ailments and thinning of the semen.

Bath Temperature

The most important practice to follow before the morning bath is to allow skin temperature to equalize with air temperature in the bathroom. Sudden changes in temperature create disturbances in the system and should always be avoided. The body temperature and room temperature should be equal — as should the temperature of the shower or bath.

·Skin temperature increases following sleep, defecation, intercourse, food, exercises and massage. It is therefore necessary to allow a lapse of about 30 minutes for the skin temperature to become acclimated. Once body temperature normalizes, the bath may be taken.

Both the Indian and Greek medical systems praise the virtues of lukewarm water for bathing. To give a specific temperature range for all persons would be foolish. Some individuals have an excessive amount of heat in their systems (especially *pitta*-dominated people) and require a compensating amount of cold, while others have too much cold (the *kapha*-dominated) and would do well to take warmer baths. The introductory chapter on dietary principles discusses these physiological types in detail — for now it can be said that "cold-blooded" people need warmer baths than do the "hot-blooded".

Those troubled by excessive heat should bathe with water slightly below air temperature, while those who suffer from cold should use water just slightly warmer. In no cases should water be so hot as to cause condensation on the bathroom mirror (an excellent gauge) or to make goosebumps to appear on the body.

The best indicator of proper bath temperature is one's state following the towelling-off. If one feels refreshed, invigorated, enthused and inspired, the bath temperature is proper.

Water cooler than room temperature is especially indicated in two cases: hot summer months, and when one has lost energy through excessive, prolonged sexual indulgence. Cool and cold water baths are beneficial for those with scalp disorders and habitual dullness and drowsiness.

One can experiment with his own organism by bathing in warm-to-hot water for 15 successive days; lukewarm for an equal period, followed by fortnights of cool and cold. By this practice one quickly establishes what is best for his own system.

If one suffers from headaches, dullness or drowsiness, bath temperature should be reduced. Temperature can be considered proper when one feels fresh, energetic, eats and digests properly, has a clean bowel movement and a healthy body.

Bathing Procedures

Before entering a shower or tub, first wash the feet, then the hands — and then pour bath temperature water (if a cool or cold bath) over the head. The first two steps remove the greatest accumulation of dirt and bad chemicals, while the latter prevents headaches.

If the water temperature is at variance with air temperature, slowly expose the body, starting with feet and gradually progressing upwards.

If one has applied oil or oil-flour paste to his body beforehand, no additional cleansing agents are necessary. But if such is not the case, organic cleansing products are always preferable to detergents, soap cakes and shampoos. With few exceptions, commercial soaps contain caustic lye. The skin absorbs chemicals through the pores, and anything which it contacts reaches all the organs. Additionally, virtually all cleansers — synthetic and organic — remove vital oils from the skin, scalp and hair — which the body must then replace at the cost of additional energy.

If one does use a commercial cleanser, he should apply mustard or olive oil to the skin before dressing to alleviate dryness.

Singing or humming in the shower or tub proves a most beneficial practice. Humming especially helps to equalize body temperature.

As one bathes, he should rub the body in an even rhythmic manner — greatly facilitated by singing or humming. Bathroom singers are famous in India — a country where one who does not sing is immediately besieged with concerned inquiries about his state of health. Humming and singing disappear only in states of physical or mental turmoil.

Tub or shower: which is better? The main disadvantage of tub baths is the feeling of relaxation which may easily lead to sleep — which raises body temperature. Otherwise tub baths are good for patients with abdominal complaints and piles. The shower prevents sleep and is generally a better method of bathing.

After The Bath

After stepping from the tub or shower the body should immediately be dried. A brisk rubbing with a Turkish-type towel (always cotton) increases circulation and energizes the system.

Fresh clothing should always be worn following the bath, otherwise one puts on old vibrations and smells. It is impossible to feel as comfortable in clothes which have been worn and not washed as one feels in fresh, crisp clothing. If one must wear clothing which is not fresh, the underwear at least should be fresh and clean.

These articles should not be used more than one day without washing.*

When Not To Bathe

Daily bathing is essential in almost all cases for maintenance of good health, but there are exceptions.

Patients of fever should avoid bathing. Ear infections preclude bathing, as well as gastric upset, and constipation.

Bathing should also be avoided when left or both nostrils work.

Miscellaneous Personal Hygiene

In addition to the practices discussed in preliminary cleansing, there are several other procedures which should be followed to insure the most effective operation of the bodily system.

WASHING THE FEET: Before and after taking food, one should wash the feet as well as hands and face. Similarly, after returning from a journey, long or short, one should immediately take off shoes and socks and allow the feet to equalize with air temperature (open sandals whenever possible are the best footgear). After feet have reached room temperature, wash them with cool water. This practice increases vitality, and creates good feelings in the heart. Washing the feet three or four times daily is very beneficial: before and after meals and before sleep. Washing before going to bed aids sound sleep.

HAIR CUTS: Men should have their hair cut weekly

---

* The practice of not wearing underclothing has become fashionable of late. This is very unhealthy and unattractive. Underclothes insulate against sudden changes of temperature and conserve energy within the system — as well as keeping bad smells at a minimum and providing proper support to genital and breast tissues.

— or at least monthly. Women, however, should not cut their hair because they need the extra solar energy received by the hair during the course of the day. Both men and women should keep hair clean and never allow it to become dry.

SHAMPOOING: Hair should always be kept clean and full of natural oils. Dryness causes a loss of electrical energy, weakens memory and encourages fantasy. A mixture of mustard oil and chickpea flour applied to the hair just before showering cleans the oils. Yogurt also serves as an excellent natural hair cleaner. In no cases should commercial preparations be used.

COMBING THE HAIR: This practice keeps the upper part of the head free from dirt, and frequent combing (many times daily) benefits both general health and eyesight by drawing the flow of electrical energy to the upper portion of the head (just as stroking a cat generates electrical charges). This practice of frequent combing is especially recommended for the elderly.

Combs of wood are good for the eyesight, horn for the hair, silver for the heart and gold for the brain. Having one's hair combed by children is also extremely beneficial. The practice of running one's finger through his hair is frowned on as it raises sexual energies and stimulates fantasies by increasing pituitary gland function. If no comb is available, pat the hair instead.

NAILS: Fingernails should be trimmed and cleaned to provide proper growth and the most pleasing visual effect.

Because the nature of energy on the planet varies from day to day, certain times are more beneficial than others for performing these personal hygiene functions. Hindus believe that men should shave on Mondays, Wednesdays and Fridays only; women should trim excess body-hair at five-day intervals. Both sexes should avoid cutting any body or head hair on Tuesdays, Thursdays and weekends. Trimming the nails should be done on the same days as shaving.

Shaving or cutting hair on Tuesdays is said to result in injury to the body; on Thursdays, loss of job or money; Saturdays, sufferings and ailments to progeny; Sundays, fear of humiliation. In addition, one should avoid washing laundry on Thursday or washing the hair with other than pure clean water.

For The Eyes

The eyes are a delicate and sensitive sense organ, easily injured and weakened — and healed only with time and care. The greatest enemy of good eyesight is sudden changes in temperature, such as a sun bath followed by splashing cold water in the eyes or a sauna bath followed by a cold shower. Squinting and straining to see distant objects also impairs vision, as does sleeping in the day and resisting the natural urge to sleep at night. (For this latter reason, one who is conducting a sleep-fast should close his eyes to relax them at those moments when he feels awake and alert, and walk or move around when feeling sleepy. Under normal circumstances one should not sleep fast more than twice in a lunar month, Darkest Night and Full Moon.)

Excessive crying spoils the vision, as do sorrow, anger and emotional suppression. Excessive sexual indulgence, physical injury, consuming too much vinegar and citrus fruit, and eating an excess of gas-producing food also causes visual problems. One who resists the natural urges to urinate, defecate, belch and cough also suffers eye problems. Excessive vomiting and the suppression of vomiting both lead to eye problems; as does roaming in dusty places, standing near hot water (exposing the eyes to steam), exposure to toxic fumes, suppression of crying and disturbance of bile.

In general, the eyes should always be saved from smoke, bad air, excessive crying, excessive use of intoxicants (so that the eyes become "bloodshot" and the eye loses its natural glaze and ability to reflect light).

One should never try to see minute objects without the aid of a lens, nor should one write in a very small script. One who keeps his hair dry and without oil also troubles his eyes, as does one who reads at sunset or in the late evening. Reading by artificial light or by kerosene causes eyestrain. Riding on speedy vehicles should be avoided whenever possible, as the rapidly moving air dries the eyes.

There are also many ways of helping preserve and improve the vision. Seeing green objects is excellent, which is one reason why working or walking in a garden or forest helps the eyes. One may also massage his head with different compounds according to the season: sandalwood paste in hot weather, mustard oil in cold weather, and black sesame and coconut oils in the moderate seasons. Application of sandalwood paste to the area between the eyebrows also helps the vision, especially when camphor and saffron are added to the paste (the nerves absorb both the volatile chemicals from the camphor and the iodine from the saffron, directly stimulating and nourishing the optic nerve). Whenever the eyes feel tired or strained, one should wash the mouth three times with cold water — a great preventive device.

The top of the cranium should be massaged daily with oil to keep the vision intact, or at least two or three times weekly on a regular basis. Oil massage should also be given immediately following a hair-cut. But applying *ghee* (clarified cow's butter) at the top of the head while eating a small amount of *ghee* and rock sugar candy, one greatly benefits his eyes. If the *ghee* is prepared from fresh, sweet butter, the practice of massage combined with eating a small amount of the *ghee* will placate disorders of bile and blood, increase *ojas* and semen in the system, impart strength to the whole system and give both fresh, useable protein and natural vitality. Yet the *ghee* prepared in this way is still cold in nature and beneficial to the system.

There is also a direct link between the feet and the eyes through two primary spinal nerves. Wearing shoes which do not allow the feet to breathe impairs function of these nerves and spoils the eyes (as does exposing the feet to a fire or other kinds of excessive heat). By keeping the feet clean, eyesight is aided. Massage of the feet with clay, mud, and henna pastes also improves the vision. Henna is especially good, but only for use in warm and hot weather because of its strong cooling power. By application of oils and pastes to the feet, coupled with a gentle massage, one waters the plant of good vision and insures proper eyesight in later life.

A powder of three dried fruits (amla, harrar and bahera) each in equal measure when kept in silver or copper container overnight (one teaspoon of powder to a cup of water) can be used in the morning to wash the eyes. This solution is the greatest medicine for the eyesight against the natural effects of aging. Washing the head once a week with this same solution will also improve the vision, as will a bath in the paste made of dried amla fruit.

A paste of black sesame seeds massaged into the head before bathing will improve eyesight and quell gastritis. Using snuff once or twice monthly also helps vision by purging the sinuses and the frontal lobes of the brain. Swimming in clear, untreated water with open eyes is also very beneficial (but this should *never* be done in chlorinated water. The hairs of the nose should never be plucked as this puts a great strain on the nerves and muscles of the face and troubles the vision.

Reading by the light of a lamp fuelled by mustard oil or *ghee* is great for the eyesight.

In the process of aging, the heat inside the body gradually diminishes. This, in turn, affects the operation of all systems, but the eyes in particular. One who follows some or all of the practices outlined above can, if he starts before his 40th birthday, save his vision for the length of his life, barring severe illness or accident.

A final preparation for the eyes is *kajul,* the soot (lampblack) made from a flame fuelled either by *ghee* or mustard oil. This powder, when applied to the edge of the lower eyelid, absorbs excessive light and provides a means of insuring that no destructive intensities of light can reach the eyes.

Sitting By A Fire

Whenever possible one should devote the first part of the early morning to sitting by a natural wood fire with his chest facing the flames. Fire contains electrically charged ions which fill the immediate atmosphere and enter into the system through the nostrils and lungs, conveying vital energy to all portions of the organism.

By facing the fire the muscles of the chest and the heart are suffused by the warmth, promoting regular breathing and a slow, regular heartbeat. The heat and electrical ions also enable the blood to become thin and thus penetrate the tissues more effectively. This whole process stimulates the proper flow of gases in the system.

Fire is the equivalent of sunlight in a form which is very beneficial and easily utilized — and a wood fire is best. Saints in India, soon after rising, kindle fires and sit for an hour before their morning worship. They know that plants, through the process of photosynthesis, convert sunlight into a useable form (firewood).

All nourishment comes from the sun. All foods are formed by plants at the base of the life chain. Even meat-eating animals consume sunlight which has been converted to flesh by herbivorous animals. And all plants create nutriments from the chemicals of the soil, water, and carbon dioxide from the air. These three elements combined together with sunlight create the very tissues of life.

Thus firewood is stored solar energy, and fire releases the light and energy of the wood into the atmosphere.

Six

The Meaning Of Meditation

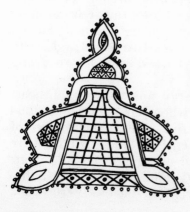

The most precious moments in a man's life extend from the completion of morning cleansing to the minutes just following the dawning of the new day. The actions he performs within the space of these few minutes register indelibly on the organism, determining the course of the succeeding 24 hours.

Purified within and without, the system has been rendered a blank slate.

One who uses these moments wisely can erect an energy field capable of shielding out all but the strongest of negative vibrations — and those which do penetrate disturb him far less than one who has not well used the golden minutes of the morning.

One who has performed the morning waking and cleansing practices insures that his system is free of wastes and toxins, and the changes produced by the natural changes in the blood create far more positive effects than sleep.

But the process does not end here ...

In sleep the body's energies are dispersed throughout the system, revitalizing each strand of muscle fibre. Through the mechanism of sleep the energies drained by the actions of the day are restored by the primordial healing process.

But there are two organs whose work never ceases, heart and brain.

What of the heart? This untiring fist-sized mass of tissue works incessantly, pumping life's blood throughout the system. In anger it beats faster, as it does in all states of extreme arousal. In sleep, reverie and relaxation it slows. But heart never stops. So long as there is life, the heart must work.

And what of the brain? What of this complex of nerve tissues which, waking and sleeping, directs and controls the actions of the organism? The brain never sleeps. During the night, as the body relaxes, the brain continues its commands. In addition, it must process the sensory overload of the previous day — discharging unfulfilled desires through the mechanism known as dreaming.

Sleep, massage and exercise relax and stimulate the body back into proper tone. But what can be done for heart and brain? These two organs safeguard the human organism so long as life exists. If either is destroyed, death comes instantaneously.

Heart and brain, working together in harmony, are the embodiments of the preservative force in the human system. Yet even the Preserver needs rest, relaxation — a few moments when its load can be lessened. So too do these organs need rest — so that each and every cell can be permeated and charged with life-renewing energies.

This concentration of energy and slowing of heart and brain cycles occurs only when one experiences total absorption in the moment and total concentration of energy. In this state, all tensions and defences are dropped — and the liberated energy rushes into heart and brain. Breath rate slows, and with it the rhythm of the heart. The brain is centred on one perception, all others being ignored. Brainwaves slow, synchronize and disharmonic patterns vanish.

In these moments there exists nothing other than that which is perceived — the one object of concentration. No extraneous thoughts flow, no disturbing signals from body are registered. One is no longer concerned with anything, for concern implies separation — and in this state no separation exists. There is no desire to speak, no desire to move, no desire to think, no desire to feel — no desire at all.

But how does one attain this state?

Anyone who is reading this book has experienced this state at least once, for only the taste of this limitless bliss can lead one on the path towards self-change and evolution.

The cause might have been anything — relaxation following the completion of a long and arduous project, a meeting with a new person, a musical composition, a majestic view, a penetrating book, a severe illness, a drug — any of these might have been the trigger.

Whatever the cause, one who has known this experience remains forever changed, just as one's whole way of seeing the world changes after the first unassisted steps of childhood. And from this moment life has but one meaning, one goal; how to get back, how to regain that once-felt bliss. Vainly one repeats the actions which brought him there the first time, but to no avail. It first happened, he soon realizes, precisely because he was *not* seeking it, for in the act of consciously seeking the state of egolessness the ego becomes inextricably involved.

Vainly one tries to render the mind empty, a void. But the mind is not so easily controlled. For a moment now and then it seems as if one is almost there, perched just on the brink — and then the very realization that one is almost there draws consciousness back into the world of distractions. One is reminded of the time he went somewhere, or the pleasant dinner he had, or the new shoes, or the cat scratching at the door, or the unpaid bills — the list is endless, one soon discovers.

The more the fantasies come, the greater becomes the sense of frustration — and the greater the frustration, the further away the state one is seeking.

Until this moment, meditation has been a term without personal value — an "in" word floating periodically in the stream of consciousness. But still only a word. Now it returns, carrying with it the glistening promise that here might just be the key to unlocking that stubborn door within one's own mind — the doorway leading to ineffable rapture.

Once meditation establishes itself in the conscious mind, one has begun a long and difficult search. He encounters scores of books, tracts, magazines, records, tape recordings, pictures and even machines — all virtually guaranteed to offer him the *only* sure path to enlightenment.

But in all these there is a depressing sameness, a few overworked catch words and a great deal of mystical verbiage. Nowhere does he discover a real understanding of meditation. Few works stress the importance of cleansing the body, few stress the importance of rising before dawn. Few, indeed, even give the reasons for meditating only when relaxed and on an empty stomach.

There are teachers, but all too often they demand total subservience — making of their followers mindless automations who bear a discomforting resemblance to troops of soldiers.

Tantric Meditation

The purpose of work on the self is to create light and to embody the Truth in every thought and action. To create light is to dispel darkness, to destroy occultism and mysticism. Occult literally means concealed, hidden from light; mystical means hidden, mysterious.

The ancient science of *Tantra Yoga* offers empirically

proven methods of centring energy, techniques which when practised through time, promise the slow but genuine evolution of psychic energy.

Foremost among these practices is *tratak*.

The word *tratak* comes from the Sanskrit *trut*, the act of coming to tears. *Tratak* is a practice used to excite the energy level of the brain and to concentrate all mental energies at one point, one centre of visual attention. Although in popular Western usage *tratak* has come to mean simple candle meditation, the concept conveys far more than concentration on a flame alone.

Any source of visual input, near or far, on which the meditator can direct his gaze without blinking until tears begin to flow may be used as the object of concentration. *Tratak* is the process of creating a state of one-pointedness by centring attention through the eyes.

Tratak consists of three fundamental stages: calming the system through regulation of breath; centring visual attention on one object or point until tears flow; and closing the eyes and visualizing the object as it appears in the form of a retinal after-image: relaxation, concentration and meditation.

Relaxation is the process of creating a uniform flow of energy throughout the system by regulating the cycle of breath. Concentration is the process of directing all conscious energies towards a single object of sense perception. Withdrawing the sense organs inward and opening the self to the experience of inner perception is the practice of meditation.

Mind and The Senses

To understand *tratak* it is first necessary to have a firm grasp on the nature of mind itself, and of the currents of energy which operate in human consciousness. Yogis understand mind as one of the four attributes of consciousness: *manas, buddhi, ahamkara* and *chitta*. *Manas* is mind; *buddhi* is intellect; ego is *ahamkara*, being — the essence of man — is *chitta*.

Whatever happens transpires within a continuum of actions and interactions. The sense organs are the windows of the mind, of *manas*. Each message from the phenomenal world passes through these windows for presentation by the mind to *buddhi* intellect. Intellect is the adviser who stores all that which has happened in past experience and all possibilities the future holds. He is conscious of the positive and negative aspects of anything the mind presents, and always perceives through a three-dimensional framework of past, present and future.

Like an honest friend, *buddhi* guides the human organism while remaining unattached to anything, a friendly but unbiased judge.

Ego is that which identifies and acts. While intellect judges, *ahamkara* acts on these judgments — denying that which is unacceptable and acting out that which is acceptable. Ego is the self-concept, that which creates a sense of separation from other beings. Ego is the faculty for extending being into the phenomenal world.

Chitta is the feeling self, the core of being. All the actions of the ego register on the *chitta*. Acts which are in accord with this Essence, or inner nature, produce feelings of bliss. Contrary actions create feelings of pain and displeasure. *Chitta* is beyond the senses, and beyond evaluation and identification.

Energy, in the form of light, sound, smell, taste or touch, reaches the eyes, ears, nose, taste buds or touch receptors. This incoming energy excites the sense organ starting a process which culminates in the brain. These incoming currents cause detectable changes in the function of the organism.

Sense perceptions energize the mind, and a duplicate of the original stimulus is presented to the intellect and ego within the skull, within the tissues of the brain itself. Energy from outside the organism penetrates the brain (the gross manifestation of mind) through the sense organs and nervous system, to be manifested as changes in consciousness. Perceptions of the outside world are in reality events within the mind/brain itself, triggered by an external source of energy. Thus, for example, what one actually hears is not the external sound, but electromagnetic pulses of the nervous system vibrating in resonance with the external sound — *not the external stimulus itself.*

One is continually surrounded by objects of sensory stimulation, and the act of centring attention on any one source can often be accomplished only with great difficulty. Other sources compete with the object of concentration, causing lapses in the attention span. And it is through the mind that all distractions come into consciousness.

One is concentrating on writing a letter when a motion is seen out of the corner of one eye. Mind has presented a sense perception to the intellect. Intellect now registers the motion as of indeterminate origin, and of unknown possible consequences to the organism. Ego, concerned with the presence of the unknown and seeking to make a positive identification, directs the head and eyes to turn towards the source of motion. It is, one discovers, merely the wind blowing a curtain. Pleased and relaxed, one returns to the task of writing.

In this mundane sequence, all the four elements are clearly visible. Mind presented the blur of motion to intellect. Intellect gave an "unknown" signal to ego. Ego, not content with uncertainty, strove to make the identification by commanding the body to act. The feeling self, once the identification was made, registered relief.

From the original task one was distracted into a long and involved process, one which shattered the original sequence of thought. To return to the letter now necessitates a moment of reflection and recollecting, of "gathering one's wits".

Sense perceptions are presented to the intellect for evaluation, and then passed on to ego for action. Intellect is the function of consciousness which scans the raw content of sense perceptions, looking for aspects which correlate with past experiences. Each of these aspects is then integrated into a single judgment, and on the basis of this judgment the ego acts. The ego attaches to sense objects, desiring to attain for itself those which have been deemed necessary for maintaining or extending the identity.

The very act of evaluation, coupled with the action which follows, is a process of projecting conscious energy outward in the form of attachment to sense objects. This, the phenomenon of desire, accounts for the daily depletion of conscious (psychic) energy.

One receives energy from the material world in the form of sense perceptions. This energy is then projected back onto the material world in the form of desires and attachments. Normally this flow of energy back and forth through the gates of mind reaches an equilibrium — as much as one receives, one gives back.

But to attain the state of meditation, to work consciously to raise the level of being, one must raise the level of energy present within his own mind. One must begin to perceive the world without attachments, without value judgments, without desires. And to reach this state the energies in the organism must first become one-pointed. This, the state of concentration, is the necessary precursor to meditation itself.

Tratak induces this single-mindedness by focusing awareness on a flame or a black circle. After slowing and synchronizing his breath, the meditator gazes into the object of concentration with both eyes.

Tratak induces the state of single-pointedness by first stilling and harmonizing the breath, and then by providing a fixed source of sensory input at which one gazes, both eyes sharply focused, until the mind frees itself of all external distractions.

A flame or black circle is customarily used, for either of these objects may be easily perceived without attaching valuations — enabling the meditator to still the flow of thoughts which often begins with the perception of a sense object. The lens of the eye, in turn, focuses the image on the retinal surface where it is passed through the optic nerves to the occipital lobes of the brain. All energy is thus focused on one point, incoming and outgoing. A closed loop is formed.

When tears flow, the meditator closes his eyes and visualizes the spot or flame internally, where it appears as an afterimage on the retina — the surface of the brain's optic nerve. The eyes are brought to one internal point, just slightly above the centre of the browline. The eyes are now directed to the plexus (juncture) of the three nerves considered most important in yoga physiology. This is the plexus activated by the pineal gland.

The pineal, located in the centre of the brain between the two hemispheres, is the only gland in the human body which is receptive to light. For this reason, it has been called the *third eye* in traditional spiritual literature. It is this gland which converts the energy of light into the electromagnetic frequencies used to govern the operation of the entire glandular system.

The pineal literally feeds on light, and denied proper input normally atrophies by the age of 16. Light is then the food of the pineal, and denied its sustenance the organ withers. For this reason traditional Indian families keep an oil lamp burning in an infant's nursery at all times during the first crucial 40 days of life. And while most forms of meditation are expressly prohibited for children, *tratak* is prescribed at a very early age.

Yoga has long recognized the significance of the pineal, and of the necessity of disciplines to prevent the atrophy of the "master gland" of the body.

Fortunately, the pineal never completely withers. It remains always sensitive to light, and with proper stimulation can redevelop. By concentrating all frequencies of the visual light spectrum into one compact but not-too-intense source — as with the flame of a lamp fuelled by clarified butter — light and heat can be conveyed to the pineal through the optic nerves. Regular practice of *tratak* on a flame initiates the gradual process of redevelopment. When proper pineal function is restored — virtually impossible without some form of regular concentration on light — light is converted into electrical energy and sent from the pineal under conscious direction to the other glands of the endocrine system through the nerve junction in the region of the forehead where the eyes are upturned both in meditation and unconsciousness. When one is conscious and experiencing the flow of energy through this plexus, one experiences intense bliss. This moment, when the energy is first brought under conscious control, has been called the *opening of the third eye*.

With full pineal function restored, the body gains a new balance. Nerve energy flows evenly through both halves of the organism. Neither electrical nor magnetic currents predominate. In this state the central passage of the spinal cord opens and energy flows upward through the spine into the brain. It is this upward rush of energy which is experienced as bliss, the state which the meditator knew long before — and which drove him to seek the disciplines of self-evolution.

The opening of the pineal takes time. What took years to wither does not miraculously regenerate overnight. *Tratak* is a discipline of *yoga* requiring regular and persistent practice. But there are immediate effects as well: enhanced ability to concentrate, greater awareness of the visual realm, a more centred and relaxed state of mind — and the positive feelings which flow from the knowledge that one has at last discovered a means of elevating consciousness.

Concentration on the flame opens the door to one-pointedness —and all potentials are but the extensions of a single point. Hindu scriptures say that one who practises *tratak* regularly develops the faculties of intuition and imagination. Past, present and future appear with equal clarity in a state of pure rapture, beyond all limitations and attachments.

Practice of Tratak

The meditator's first need is a quiet part of the house where he can practice regularly. Regularity of practise is essential to accomplishing his goal. The meditator should sit on a skin (*yogis* prefer tiger or deer), a straw mat or a woollen blanket. This is his *asana* and serves to prevent discharge of the body's electrical energy into the earth (concentration brings this energy to the head, and its loss would hinder meditation). The *asana* should be used solely for meditation and not changed from day to day. Through the passage of time, objects used as part of the practice of meditation absorb the energies of the meditator. This energy helps him enter and maintain the meditative state. Similarly, no one else should be allowed to use or handle the *asana* to keep the vibrational pattern intact.

One should always sit in the posture best suited to one's self, in which one feels the most comfortable and the fewest possible distracting bodily sensations. *Yogis* prefer the *sidha asana* (where right leg crosses over left, with the left heel positioned midway between the anal and genital regions, maintaining a gentle pressure on the base of the spine) or the cross-legged lotus posture. The spine must be kept vertical to the floor at all times. If one experiences discomfort, a pillow may be used as a seat on top of the *asana*. This should be a cotton or wool pillow — never a synthetic fabric. Knees should always touch the floor.

The meditator now closes his right nostril and inhales for one time unit, holds the breath for four and exhales for two units through his left nostril, then reverses the procedure and breathes through the right with the left closed. This cycle is maintained until one is able to breathe through both nostrils simultaneously, a process which creates a state of balance in the breath and aids meditation.*

The meditator lights the *ghee* lamp which he has positioned eleven inches in front of his face at eye-level. He takes five deep breaths, retaining the last — stopping the breath at the nostrils, not locking the lungs. These should be done so slowly that the sound of breath is not heard. With lungs full, he opens his eyes, smiles and gazes at the midpoint of the flame without blinking until tears begin to flow from both eyes. The duration between starting the gaze and the flow of tears may well be beyond the meditator's capacity to retain the air in his lungs, especially at the beginning of practice. If one must breathe, then one does so deeply and slowly, causing no rapid changes of pressure in the lungs. Under no circumstances, however, does he allow his eyelids to close until tears flow from both eyes. He smiles always while gazing at the flame. This relaxes the muscles of the throat and jaw.

When the tears begin to flow, one closes the eyes and turns them upward to the third eye, just above the centre of the browline, as the lungs are emptied. One can see the flame as a retinal after-image at the point the attention is centred. As long as the image remains, the eyes remain closed and turned upward. One may begin to see recognizable forms within the image. If so, they are observed without attachment, without attempting to change or eliminate them.

When the image vanishes, the meditator inhales and holds the air in his lungs. Still retaining the air he rubs his face; first stroking out from the third eye along the browline to the temples, then working outward from the root of the nose along the muscles at the base of

---

* Normally during the course of the day either one nostril or the other predominates in the breathing process. When this flow is equalized and one breathes evenly through both nostrils the body's energies are balanced. In this state energy can flow upward through *shushumna*, the central passage of the spinal column, to the brain.

the eyesockets. On the same inhalation, the meditator locks his hands behind his neck and pushes backward with the top of his head, stretching and straightening the spine. Lastly, still on the same breath, he moves his hands down over the heart, left over right, with palms inward.

Now the meditator exhales, totally exhausting the air from his lungs, and meditates on his heart so long as he need not inhale. When the breath must again come, the eyes are kept closed for the space of five or more deep breaths, which helps to stabilize body temperature.

Tratak is now complete. The meditator opens his eyes to any direction but south, preferably seeing the green of a living plant or a freshly cut flower. It is important that one not see the flame again for ten minutes, to preserve the effects of meditation.

Because concentration on a candle flame increases the amount of heat and light energy in the eyes, cleansing and cooling the eyes after *tratak* is of special importance. After the meditator has opened his eyes he should either wash his eyes with rosewater or drink water through his nostrils, spitting it out through the mouth. One can use a drop of rosewater in each eye; or take lukewarm water, slightly salted and with a little *ghee* added, and inhale through the nostrils. Both cool and cleanse the eyes.

After cleansing the eyes, the meditator sits down quietly in his posture and closes his eyes, moving them from left to right, right to left, and up and down. This discharges the tension built up in resisting the impulse to blink and stabilizes the meditator in his state of relaxation.

Times To Meditate

To be most effective, *tratak* must be practised daily at a regular time. The best times to practise are those which synchronize the meditator's daily life with the larger cycles of the planet and cosmos.

The mood of the planet changes dramatically at the times of sunrise and sunset. This change, which begins about 30 minutes before the sun touches the horizon and lasts for an hour, also produces marked changes in blood chemistry.

In addition, at the exact moment the sun touches the horizon, the organism automatically breathes through both nostrils simultaneously. This is the state in which energy can flow up the *shushumna* passage of the spinal cord to the brain, the same state induced by the alternate nostril breathing technique described earlier. During *shushumna* body chemistry is balanced. Because both nostrils are working, the temperature of the air in the sinus cavities is equalized. The temperature of both hemispheres of the brain is balanced, and metabolism (the rate at which energy can be consumed) is equal. Both hemispheres can now function in synchronization. This is the ideal state for meditation.

The meditator should always make use of these planetary cycles and energy changes in his organism. This enables one to live more harmoniously with the natural flow of life, and is the reason why meditation at sunrise and sunset has been prescribed by all the world's religions in one form or another.

One should always prepare for meditation by bathing the body (a cool shower is best) and changing into clean clothing, preferably loose-fitting and of natural fibres. This purifies the body and stimulates the flow of energy through the system. Pores are opened and there are no body odours lingering on the clothing.

Tratak should never be practised more than twice in the course of any given day. Sunrise is the most important and beneficial of all times to practise. At sunrise particularly, there is a tremendous increase in energy. Plants and animals spring into life, refreshed and rejuvenated. Sunset practice is also beneficial, but is not essential.

Meditation at the darkest hour of the night, midway between sunset and sunrise, is prescribed by Hindu scriptures as the time to meditate when faced with a seemingly insoluble problem. Practise *tratak* for 40 consecutive nights and the answer will be found, *tantrics* say.

Regularity of practice and sunrise *tratak* are essential.

The Witness Consciousness

Meditation on the flame of a lamp produces a state of mind called the witness consciousness. This witness of the self is ageless and timeless, that essence which survives all transformations of personality, all emotional storms, all changes of thought, all experience.

The witness is what remains when all social experience and heredity traits have been stripped away. What remains is common to all human experience. Called the collective unconscious in psychological literature, the witness is centred in the region of the third eye. According to *yogis,* one who centres his being here gains access to the reservoir of all human experience, past, present and future.

The individual personality construct is illusory. Thoughts change, emotions come and go. The cells of the body die by the millions between the rising of two suns, only to be replaced by equal numbers of new cells. Nothing of the body, mind, intellect or ego cannot and does not change in one fashion or another. Yet there is also a continuity of being.

The individual is a myth, an illusion, the game being played. The witness is the player. The individual is the droplet; the witness, the drop merged with the sea. *Tratak* enables the played to become the player, to erode gradually the barrier of illusion which hides the essence of being. *Tratak* burns through the myth of individual personality and restores contact with the Divine in human experience.

And in this gradual but effective process, the player can also gain valuable new insight into the energy dynamics of his own system. The daily practice of concentrating on the flame provides the clue. While gazing into the flame, one eye generally tears before the other. The meditator should always note which tears first. The right hemisphere of the brain rules the left half of the body, just as the left hemisphere rules the right half. Similarly, the left eye is linked with the right hemisphere (due to a crossing over of the optic nerves), and *vice versa*.

The right side of the body is dominated by intellect, reason, creative (electrical) energy. The left side is emotional, intuitive, receptive (magnetic). Tears in the right eye mean one is dominated by intellect, reason. Tears in the left eye mean emotions hold the reins. Simultaneous tearing shows a balance has been attained.

A change in which eye tears first may be noted from one day to the next. This indicates changes being produced by the experiences of the day. Thus the meditator can learn which activities best help him in his quest to balance his energies.

Because *tratak* works with the balance of energies in system, it is by nature *tantric*. *Tantra* is the discipline of *yoga* dealing specifically with the balance of energies.

Other Forms of Tratak

Yogis traditionally group the forms of *tratak* into three categories. First is *aantar tratak* where the meditator closes his eyes and concentrates his awareness on the third eye, heart or navel. This is also called inner *tratak* and is the final stage of the form outlined in this publication.

Second is *madhya*, or middle, *tratak*. Here the meditator gazes without blinking on a stone, metallic object, sculpture, black point, the Sanskrit character for Om, the tip of the nose or a flame.

Third is *vahiya*, outer, *tratak*, where the object of

concentration is distant. The sun, moon and planets, the top of a tree or a tower might serve as the centring point.

In a complete system, all three forms of practice are incorporated. There is always a centring object which remains in a stationary position relative to the meditator, internal or external. Having a drawing or painting on the wall opposite where one normally sits can serve as an excellent centring device at home or at work — a form of *vahiya tratak*.

Staring at the sun has cost the sight of many an aspirant. Solar radiation can burn the retina irreparably. *Tratak* on the sun should never be practised without the instruction of a *yogi* long experienced in the technique. Again, *never stare at the sun!* The retina burns quickly, before the danger becomes apparent to the conscious mind.

One can meditate on a design, a one-inch black circle on a sheet of plain white paper or a paper with a black circle which has a pinhole centre through which the meditator concentrates on a flame. But direct *tratak* on the flame of a *ghee* lamp is the only means that produces light of all visible frequencies at a level of intensity not harmful to the organism.

The meditator should always close his eyes after both tear and wash them with rosewater (or cleanse his nostrils) and not look at the flame again for ten minutes after completing the full process. By following these two simple rules, the practice of *tratak* can only help on the path to self-understanding.

The Ghee Lamp

The nature of the fuel which feeds the flame of meditation is an integral aspect of *tratak*. While any source of fire could provide the flame itself, each type of substance burned produces certain chemicals peculiar to itself. The intelligent meditator is one who uses his flame to provide chemicals which help make him more receptive to meditation.

The brain receives these chemicals as the flame converts the fuel to gaseous vapour which fills the meditator's environment and which reaches his brain through the nostrils. Most candles are made of paraffin. And when the meditator burns a paraffin candle he inhales the vapours of a petroleum distillate, part of which reaches and affects the operation of his brain cells.

According to *tantrics* a lamp fuelled by cow's butter which has been clarified by heat provides the best flame, although sesame and mustard oils are also good. The gases generated by the burning *ghee* supply more energy and vitality to the brain than any other substance. *Ghee* fumes aid the flow of energy currents coming into the mind of the meditator and thus are allies in his quest for the experience of bliss. *Yogis* also say *ghee* fumes have the power to cleanse the immediate environment of atomic radiations.

Ghee is best burned in an open lamp with a wick made fresh daily from an ordinary cotton ball, such as those used for medical and cosmetic purposes. Any small container with a slight rim to hold the melted *ghee* will suffice for the lamp (even a bottle-top will work).

To make the wick, take one-fourth of a cotton puff, lengthening slightly by pulling in the direction of the fibres. With thumb and forefinger of the left hand, hold the central body of the cotton and lengthen a short section, rolling it tightly in a clockwise direction. Now turn the cotton over and repeat the process, forming two small wicks — one on either end of the central body of the puff. Now bring the two sections together so they are parallel. Quickly and tightly twist them together, this time rolling in a counter-clockwise fashion. The body now becomes the base of the wick and should be broadened and flattened slightly, to become self-supporting and vertical. Immerse the base of the wick in the *ghee* and light after the oil has had a chance to work its way up the wick. Keep the flame at eye-level, eleven inches from the face.

To make *ghee* take any quantity of butter and melt at medium-high heat. Bubbles of a waxy yellow substance will rise to the surface, leaving a clear fluid below. Spoon off these bubbles as they appear and discard. These are the milk solids in the butter, responsible for spoilage.

When no more bubbles rise, pour the *ghee* slowly into a bottle, jar or other closed container, careful to leave the sediment of burned milk solids on the bottom of the pan. Butter clarified in this fashion can be kept indefinitely on an open shelf, and is also good for cooking. Merely melt enough daily for *tratak*.

Summary: Ten Stages of Tratak

Tratak is a form of meditation designed to raise the energy level of consciousness by concentrating the attention on a source of light or a point. The *ghee* lamp is considered the most beneficial object of concentration. This process of concentration and meditation on light can be divided into ten stages:

1. Sit comfortably on a woollen, skin or straw mat *asana* shortly before sunrise and sunset.
2. By alternate nostril breathing or waiting until the moment *shushumna* starts naturally, get both nostrils working simultaneously.
3. Hold the breath in the lungs and, with a smile, gaze into the midpoint of the flame of a *ghee* lamp which has been placed at eye-level, eleven inches from the face. Breathe if necessary, but always deeply, slowly, inaudibly.
4. When tears flow, empty lungs and close the eyes.
5. Bring the eyes to the third eye and concentrate on the after-image until it vanishes, breathing slowly and deeply.
6. Fill lungs, hold breath and rub face. Stroke outward

from third eye along browline to temples, then from root of the nose out along base of eyes to temples.

7. On same breath, lock fingers behind neck and push back with top of head to loosen and straighten spine.

8. Exhaust air from lungs as hands move palms inward to rest over the heart, left hand over right. Meditate on heart as long as lungs remain empty.

9. Returning to original posture, take five deep breaths and open eyes in any direction but south to stare for a few seconds at a flower or green plant. Do not see *ghee* lamp flame for ten minutes.

10. Cleanse eyes, either with a drop of rosewater in each eye or by drinking warm saltwater through the nostrils, spitting it out through the mouth. After cleaning, close eyes and exercise them by moving several times left to right, right to left and up and down.

Seven

Diet: Why Vegetarianism?

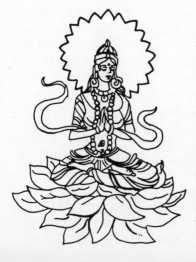

Concern with the possibility of living a harmonious life, free from anxiety and tension, inevitably leads one to a consideration of diet — specifically, the issue of vegetarianism.

The virtues of flesh consumption are continually extolled by spokesmen for public schools and state and federal agricultural departments. From childhood one is instilled with the belief that meat is essential, one of the "four pillars" of the balanced diet, necessary for good health and well-being. And yet there are millions who apparently live full and vigorous lives without ever tasting a morsel of it.

One who is considering this basic dietary question soon encounters a welter of conflicting claims and counter-claims. When condensed to essential form, the arguments in favour of meat consumption rest on the issue of "dietary necessity", while the counter-arguments are based on the harmfulness of toxins found in meat and the emotional resistance to killing another animate being for food.

The first question which

must be raised in any consideration of diet is: Why eat in the first place? The answer appears obvious at first — one eats in order to live. But witness the well-documented cases of *yogis* who have not touched any food or drink for years. In fairness, one must add that these rare individuals spend all of their time immobile, sitting in the state of deep meditation.

Eating provides fuel for the *active* system. As long as one has to perform physical actions in the world, food is necessary to replenish the energy consumed in the process of enacting his *karmic* role. Movement expends energy, and food is energy.

Specifically, food is chemical energy taken into the system to provide cell-nurturing glucose and to provide the specific chemicals needed for building and sustaining vital tissues. And because no single food is available on a year-round basis which provides all the nutrients required by the system, one must select from a variety of foods those which meet the needs of his own unique system.

The Nature of Meat

Flesh is a dead food, often days old by the time it reaches the supermarket meat counter. In most cases, preservatives (a euphemism for chemicals which kill the micro-organisms which would otherwise develop on the surface of the dead flesh) and dyes (to mask the brown colour meat assumes with the onset of decay) are added.

Additionally, vital energy leaves the organism at death, leaving in its wake only inert chemicals. Dead food from whatever source is *tamasic* in nature — and this includes all canned fruits and vegetables. Conversely, fresh fruits and vegetables contain living energy. The seeds from such foods will germinate and grow.

Food remains in the human system for about one day before being eliminated. Thus, with the consumption of meat and canned goods, inert energy already days old is added to the system, where it must remain an additional day.

The implications of this simple fact can be readily comprehended by performing an easily-arranged experiment. Fill two glasses with room-temperature tap water. To one add a slice of fresh vegetable; to the other a bit of steak of the same size. Keep both at room temperature and observe the condition of their contents at the end of the third day.

Foods and Digestion

Carnivorous animals possess powerful stomachs and short, simple intestines, allowing foods to be processed and expelled within a 24-hour cycle. This short digestive cycle minimizes both decay and the absorption of toxic chemicals. Even so, most carnivores sleep for 10 to 24 hours following a full meal so that all energy may be concentrated on food processing. And carnivores, for the most part, eat only freshly-killed meat.

Western medical science has long known that meat-eating causes a drastic increase of toxic chemicals in the human bloodstream. Patients of severe kidney disorders are routinely placed on meatless diets. (The kidneys are the blood-purifying mechanisms which filter poisons present in the blood.) This step is taken because the increase in uric acid in the blood soars following meat intake (from cow, pig, fish or fowl) and may trigger severe coma — even death. This same chemical has been indicated as a causal factor and major irritant in arteriosclerosis and other circulatory ailments. But uric acid is not the only chemical detrimental to physical and mental well-being.

Anxiety and Meat

From a ranch or farm, the cow, sheep or pig is trucked off to a slaughter-house to be killed and butchered. The animal is suddenly yanked out of the familiar environment where its whole life has been spent, shoved into dark, cramped quarters where it must remain for hours on end — continually exposed to jarring vibrations, sudden starts and stops, radical temperature changes, and disturbing sounds as it travels by truck or train. Then, destination reached, men armed with electric prods unload the animal and move it through a bewildering maze of ramps, chutes and chemical baths. Finally the animal arrives at the slaughter-house itself, full of the smell of blood and the sounds of hundreds of terrified animals.

Animals have emotions, as any pet owner can verify, and can experience the states of fear and panic which are produced by the process of shipping and slaughter. What physiological states accompany these emotions?

Fear is the psychophysiological response of the organism to threatening situations. Panic is fear carried to the extreme. Physiologically, presentation of a strong fear stimulus triggers a complex chain of events beginning in the brain and reaching finally every cell and fibre of the organism. Once the threat is recognized, the hypothalamus of the brain transmits a series of commands through the spinal column to nerve centres throughout the body. In the throat large quantities of thyrotopic hormone are released into the system, while the kidneys pour out a flood of adrenocorticotropic hormone. These in turn trigger a programmed series of responses throughout the body.

Facial and limb muscles gorge with blood drawn from the now constricted vessels of skin and digestive system. The spleen contracts, pouring out a flood of white corpuscles and platelets into the bloodstream. Heartbeat, blood pressure, and breath rate soar, and every muscle stands tensed. The liver forces out a stream of blood sugar to feed the extreme demands made by the aroused system. Nostrils expand to take in the maximum amount of air, and the eyes dilate to take in the widest possible range of visual stimuli. The abdominal gases move downward, forcing stool and urine from the system and lightening the organism.

The chemicals which produce these reactions in animals produce the same reactions in human beings. Adrenalin from the horse is used medicinally to produce the same results in man as does human adrenalin.

In the state of hyperarousal every cell of the body is filled with these chemicals, which remain after the rendering process. Regular consumption of the flesh of animals increases the presence of these same chemicals in the human system, where they produce exactly the same results — though on a modified scale. The body of a meat-eating individual is continually in a state of drugged hyperarousal, creating chronic tension, anxiety and feelings of insecurity and confusion.

With the chemicals of arousal already present in excess in the system, natural arousal is masked. One is no longer capable of responding naturally to different situations. The excess energy present in the system demands release — whether through sex, drugs or the sublimated violence of television, films and print. One simply becomes perplexed, confounded and out of touch with his true inner feelings and urges. The ever-present subtle sensation of fear created by the chemicals creates fear-of-self, psychological repression.

In no other era has meat been so plentifully available. With the increased abundance brought on with the age of electricity and refrigeration has come a corresponding increase in heart disorders, cancer, untimely deaths and a host of other ailments.

Meat was consumed previously, but never in such quantity. Also, whatever flesh was eaten before refrigeration was generally locally grown and fresh, except in major urban areas. When animals are slaughtered on the farm the level of fear-related chemicals is considerably reduced because there is no prolonged disruption of lifestyle before death.*

Carnivores and Vegetarians

Even the most casual observation of the fundamental differences between meat-eating and herbivorous animals provides valuable insight into the effects of the two dietary patterns.

First, consider the smells produced by carnivores. Compare the difference in breath smells of a cow and a cat. An attentive visit to a local zoo yields a broader sample — with the same results. The breath of meat-eating animals smells bad, far worse than that of any herbivore.

The smell of the breath is produced not only by residual particles in the mouth, but also by waste products discharged into the lungs by the incoming flow from the veins. The breath reveals the inner workings of body chemistry. The bad breath of the alcoholic emanates not from alcohol in the mouth but from the alcohol in gaseous form expelled by the lungs, indicating that the system is saturated with the drug. Similarly the breath of the carnivorous animal exudes the odours of the chemicals present in its system.

The sense of smell can readily detect another difference as well — there is a marked difference between the smells of the feces of the two groups. Cat stool is

---

* It is interesting to note the parallel between the rapid increase of tension-related disorders and two factors: mechanization and urbanization. As the lure of high wages pulled young men from rural areas to the newly industrialized cities, farm population began a slide which continues almost unabated to the present. City time is clock-oriented (9-to-5), while rural time is solar-oriented ("getting up with the chickens"). Farm people ate locally produced food, while their urban counterparts were more oriented to convenience products. Thus the move to the cities disrupted daily cycles, seasonal cycles (eating what was available locally and fresh according to season) and basic dietary patterns.

probably the most unpleasant, and cats are the strictest carnivores of all. Cow dung, on the other hand, has been burned for millennia by members of many cultures in holy rites — and forms the basic binding material in most of the forms of incense imported into the United States.

In the same vein, one can detect a major difference in the natural body odours given off by meat-eating and vegetarian humans. Provided a daily bath is taken, a vegetarian (meaning no eggs or fish) need use no deodorants or mouthwashes.

The breath rate of carnivores is fast and shallow, while herbivores breathe deeply and slowly. Fast, shallow breath in humans is associated with anxiety, tension and pain; deep, slow breath with peace, tranquillity and relaxation. Adrenalin stimulates breath, and has been prescribed by physicians for decades to stimulate heart and breath cycles — and, as noted above, adrenalin permeates the meat of animals which have been killed. In the normal individual, adrenalin overexcites and leads to chronic tension, accelerated heartbeat and rapid breath. None of these conditions is conducive to good physical and mental health.

As a group, carnivores are largely nocturnal, while vegetarians are generally diurnal — the list of possible comparisons would fill volumes. But all of these differences culminate in one fundamental understanding: the harmonious, even-paced lifestyle sought by man coincides far more closely with the nature of the herbivorous animals than with that of the flesh-eaters.

Why Carnivores?

Carnivorous animals evolved specifically to fill a niche in the ecological chain. As a general practice, they prey almost exclusively on herbivores due to the operation of two primary forces: the ability of other carnivores to defend themselves and the low level of energy available from the flesh of other meat-eaters.

Ecologists realized long ago that carnivores hold direct responsibility for maintaining the good health and well-being of the herbivores, as the animals killed by predators are almost invariably young, weak, sick or old. Only the healthiest adults survive. Hunting animals insure the process of natural selection, by which only the fittest and best adapted members survive, thus preserving the best genetic line.

Very few people have tasted the flesh of a predatory animal. The meat proves tough, stringy and difficult to digest, as well as producing unpleasant odours and tastes.

Diet and Choice

Carnivorous animals, because of their specialization, have no choice with regard to their diet. They must either eat flesh or perish — such is their natural lot. Man, however, can survive quite well without consuming flesh. The fact that millions do should be ample evidence. And if man can survive without meat, why then should he have to kill his fellow creatures for food?

By eating flesh one indirectly participates in the killing of a living being which, if given the choice, would certainly resist and run. In the case of plant food, one consumes a fruit designed for consumption by animals.

Plants become suitable foods for man in two basic circumstances: at the end of the reproductive cycle or at the end of the lifecycle. Plants rely on the consumption of their fruits for perpetuation of the species. For instance, when a tomato is eaten the seeds are not broken down by the digestive system, but pass out intact with the stool — which then becomes the source of nutrition for the seeds during the most crucial phase of growth. Most fruits and seed pods are accordingly brightly coloured and give off pleasing smells, both of which serve to attract the attention of herbivores. This is the perfect symbiosis, a biological relationship in which both sides "win." And as for most other vegetable foods, these are taken usually only when "ripe" — that is, at the end of the lifecycle.

Many self-styled "vegetarians" eat eggs to provide more protein for their diet. Eggs, like all forms of flesh, are considerably less efficient energy forms than plant food — and they are embryonic life forms as well. In America most eggs available in supermarkets are infertile, lacking in vital energy. These products have been created by chemical stimulation of the hens and will not produce a live animal. Eggs also produce foul smells in the lower tract gases.

The Source of Life

All vital energy on the planet ultimately comes from the sun. According to astronomy, even this planet itself was once a part of the sun, the father of the solar system and the source of all existence.

Of all energy sources, those which are most efficient are those closest to the source — the sun. In the production of electrical power the most efficient means promises to be thermonuclear reaction, the same process which takes place within the solar furnace.

Similarly, vegetarian food is the most efficient nutriment for the human system because plants form the base of the food chain, closest to the source of life itself. They draw carbondioxide from the atmosphere, add water and minerals from the soil — and then somehow "cook" the mixture with sunlight to produce glucose, the basic food of all living organisms. Simple logic dictates that the closer one is to the source of anything, the purer the substance will be.

All life forms ultimately depend on this process of photosynthesis, the manufacture of glucose by plants. Even carnivores ultimately rely on second-hand photosynthetic energy — first converted to flesh by the metabolism of the herbivorous prey.

What to Do?

What then is the right diet for one who is seeking to raise his personal energy level? And how can he supply proteins and other essential nutrients by living on purely vegetarian fare?

As mentioned previously, a comparison of the digestive tracts of man and carnivores reveals man to have a considerably longer intestinal system — yet shorter by an almost equal proportion than the viscera of herbivores. Apparently then the human system is not geared for eating meat, but neither is it geared for eating raw vegetables and fruits. Herbivores have long, complex tracts because considerable effort is required to break down the fibres and tissues of raw plantstuffs.

Man, however, has mastered the element of fire, thus reducing the expenditure of energy required by the intestines.

What is it that breaks down food within the digestive system if not heat, for acidity and heat are synonymous. Body heat and stomach acids provide the catalysts for the digestive reaction. Foods which are difficult to digest require more heat and a greater concentration of energy in the stomach and viscera. Thus, sick people have always been given foods which are soft and easy to digest, so that less energy is diverted from the healing process to the digestive organs.

One who is seeking to raise his energy level must inevitably conclude that digestion is one of the single greatest demands placed on the system. The more difficult a food is to digest, the more energy is required for digestion — and that much less energy is available for meditation, concentration and enjoyment.

The obvious path of least resistance is cooked vegetarian food. Heat is always required for digestion, to break down the cell walls so that the nutrients can be drawn out and absorbed by the system. This heat can come from one of two sources — the stomach or the stove.

If the energy comes from the stomach, it must first be concentrated there, meaning less energy will be available for other jobs. If, on the other hand, the heat is provided from a source outside the system — the kitchen stove — more energy remains for other tasks.

In working with energy of any form — electrical, atomic, hydraulic or psychic — the real job is to find the path of least resistance, of most work for least effort. Vegetarian food, freshly grown and cooked thoroughly, provides that path for the human diet.

And what about proteins and all those other essential dietary ingredients? All nutriments come from plants, even the ones found in beefsteak. All life has its basis in the foundation of the food chain, which is plant life. Proteins come from plants. Lentils, wheat and other grains and legumes provide more than enough protein for the human system. And a knowledge of vegetables, grains, fruits and spices can yield a richly varied and wholly satisfactory diet for anyone.

Eight

Diet :
Towards
A New
Understanding

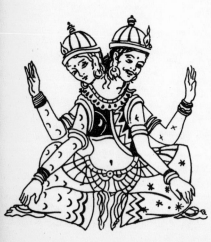

All that exists is in a state of continual vibration. Whatever we call matter is in actuality the grossest manifestation of a matter-energy continuum. Western science has classified matter into 92 naturally occurring elements (plus a score or so of synthetic laboratory products), but in India all phenomenal existence has been classed in a system of five elements.

These five elements constitute a continuum of energy from its densest, grossest vibrational level to the most subtle. This classificatory system can be most readily understood as a scale of activity and quality.

At its lowest level of vibration energy has substance (solidity), smell, taste, form, and a characteristic touch (rough, smooth, even, uneven, etc.) and — in its purest form — will produce a sound when struck. That which possesses all of these attributes is called *prithvi*, the earth element.

When excited into a higher frequency range, the earth element loses the property of solidity. The substance becomes liquid, flowing — while still retaining the properties of form (liquid assumes the form of the lowest centre of gravity), touch, and sound (produced by its motion). At this level of activity energy is called *apah*, the water element.

As the level of vibration increases, heat and light are generated by the accelerated motion. The property of liquidity vanishes, as does taste. Only touch, form and sound remain. Energy in this state is called *agnih*, the fire element.

As the speed of individual particles continues to accelerate, all form is lost and heat and light are no longer produced. Now only the properties of touch and sound remain. Solidity, liquidity and fire have disappeared. That which possesses these attributes is called *vayu*, the air element. Finally, when matter has lost all tactile qualities and is perceptible by the human organism only as sound, it has reached the most subtle level of vibration which can be apprehended by the human sensory apparatus. This is *akash*, the "ether" element.

The term "gross" can be understood as density. In the *prithvi* state energy has assumed its most dense and cohesive form — the atoms are closely packed and structured. In the *apah* state energy is less dense — the atoms are more dispersed, allowing a higher frequency rate. In the *agnih* state matter is still less cohesive, and in *vayu* all semblance of structure and cohesiveness has vanished. And at the *akash* end of the continuum the individual particles no longer exist as perceptible material — but have vibrated beyond the material plane.

In the manifest universe none of these elements exists in a pure state: all five can be found in varying proportions in any phenomenal "event". Classification is based, then, on the preponderance of a particular element or elements. These five elements, the *tattwas*, form the cornerstone of understanding for one who seeks to comprehend the Indian system of diet and medicine.

Tattwas and Physiology

The human body is composed of these same five elements. If they are present in a proper balance, the resulting state is called health. If there is prolonged imbalance, the state of disease is produced. Imbalance of one *tattwa* immediately disturbs the operation of the remaining four. Northern Indian folk medicine has as its foundation a clear understanding of the five elements and three *gunas* and the effect of their joint interaction upon the human organism.

As the three *gunas* govern the play of the whole of creation, so too do these forces govern the regulation of the human system. These three are air (gases), bile and lymph, called *vayu, pitta* and *kapha.* The harmonious balance of these three is essential for maintenance of physical and mental well-being. So long as these three remain in balance, the system digests properly, breath comes slowly and evenly, work comes easily and growth and development follow their natural and beneficial course. But with the disturbance of any one of these elements, the system becomes imbalanced — and pain and disease inevitably result.

The whole human system is governed by wind, bile and mucous, and the workings of all three are most concentrated in the region between the heart and the navel. It is this area which is the seat of most of the critical "life support" organs, those involved in the digestion, assimilation and distribution of nourishment, as well as the elimination of waste products and poisons. This is the body's workshop for self-preservation and growth, one which 24 hours a day witnesses the ceaseless interaction of the three *doshas* as they work with food material to break it down into component parts, withdraw the nutriments and then distribute these all-important chemicals throughout the system.

Disturbance of the *doshas* immediately disbalances the body's content of semen (*ojas,* see Chapter 6) and interrupts the orderly discharge of waste matter (feces, urine, perspiration and mucous). Imbalance of semen and retention of bodily wastes prove the two most powerful forces for creating disease and disorder within the body.

Because of their crucial role in regulating the human system — its growth and preservation — the three *doshas* must be understood by anyone concerned with creating balance in his organism. It is these three which are at once man's greatest friends and enemies. In balance and harmony they bring perfect health; in imbalance and disharmony it is they who cause the whole host of diseases which plague mankind.

The organisms responsible for most human disease can be found in the blood stream of anyone. Yet not everyone is sick. Disease organisms only take hold when there is an imbalance in the system which alters body chemistry and reduces the effectiveness of the system's natural antibiotic defences. These imbalances of body chemistry arise only from imbalance in the natural flow of the three *doshas*.

WIND: Vayu is the body's carrier, and like a good messenger, *vayu* can carry anything — be it the vital force needed for keeping the system alive, or chemical wastes and toxins which can destroy the delicate organs. *Rajas*-dominated, the element of wind is swift, fast, light, dry, cold and subtle in nature. Like all gases, the body air has the quality of changing its nature according to changes in temperature and pressure, and whatever it mixes with, that substance it will carry.

In whatever the disease, *vayu* is the main carrier — for it is the element of wind which distributes everything. It is the body's air which is the pneumatic power to the hydraulic pumps of the blood and lymph circulatory systems. Of the three *doshas, vayu* is thus reckoned the most important.

Vayu dwells in the stomach, waist, thighs, ears, bone and skin. Its primary seat is the stomach and intestines.

In nature it is but one, but according to location and nature of movement is divided into five sub-classes:

UDAN VAYU dwells in the throat and head region. It is with the power of this air that the second category of air, *prana,* gains the power to produce sound — speech, music and humming. When disturbed, *udan* triggers development of diseases of throat and head. Sore throat, sinus disorders, head colds, headaches, earaches and many other diseases are caused by disturbance in the operation of *udan.*

PRAN VAYU operates in the heart and lungs, and is the air which is constantly moving in and out of the nasal passages. *Prana* is the air which maintains life in the system. It is this air which helps in swallowing and bringing food and drink into the stomach. *Prana* is the primary life breath, for it is the air one breathes, and the air which brings all nourishment into the stomach. If the flow of *prana* is obstructed for an extended time, death is inevitable. Disturbances of *prana* cause hiccoughing and disorders of the lungs and breath.

SAMAN VAYU resides in the region between heart and navel, circulating primarily in the stomach and small intestines. With the help of the stomach's digestive juices, *samana* cooks the food and then separates nutrients from waste matter. When disturbed, *samana* produces a loss of stomach fire, gastritis, colic and other intestinal disorders.

APAN VAYU lives in the area between the navel and rectum. Its primary job is to expel waste materials from the system. The primary function of *apana* is to discharge the waste matter produced in the process of digestion and assimilation of food. It is also responsible for flatulation, ejaculation, conception, delivery — and defecation and urination. When disturbed, *apana* contributes to urinary and seminal disorders, hemorrhoids, constipation and a whole host of other disorders including pain and cramping of the abdomen.

VYAN VAYU keeps on circulating continuously throughout the whole body through blood vessels (as "blood gases"), the lymphatic system and the nervous system. Because it regulates the flow of all three systems, *vyana* is the most universal and significant of the airs. It is this air which takes the various nourishments from one part of the system to another, makes the blood flow, causes sweating, cleans toxins from the blood and lymph and enables the system to move in a coordinated fashion. Getting up, sitting down, pushing, pulling, opening the eyes, closing the eyes — all are done by *vyan vayu*. Disturbances in the flow of this gas result in disorders which affect the whole system.

The importance of the body's airs and gases in maintaining physical and mental health cannot be overly stressed. Air is motion itself, and without the five *vayus* the body would have no power of mobility. Neither would any of the body's internal systems be capable of functioning. If all five of these airs are disturbed simultaneously, the body meets with destruction.

BILE: Pitta is a very thin fluid, hot in nature. By itself it is dark yellow in colour, but turns bluish yellow when mixed with mucous. Light and sharp, *pitta* is hot like a chili pepper and has a greasy smooth consistency. When mixed with food in the digestive process, *pitta* assumes the characteristic sour taste one experiences when feeling "bilious". *Sattvic* in nature, it is divided into five sub-types according to location and direction of action:

PACHAK PITTA can be found in the bile duct leading to the stomach and small intestines. This agent is responsible for the digestion of the six types of food substances which reach the stomach (fatty, mucousal, well-masticated, drinkable, lightly chewed but easily digested items and foods which can be swallowed whole). By mixing with the foods, *pachak* increases the fire (acidic element) in the upper digestive tract, insuring that the food is properly "cooked" and broken down. *Pachak* then chemically separates the nutritional essence from the solid and liquid wastes, and separates the air and mucous. This is the most important of the biles, the one on which the other four depend. In large persons this compound can be found in the volume of a barley corn; while in small people it is less in quantity than a sesame seed.

RUNJAK PITTA can be found in the spleen and liver and is responsible for converting the food nutrients into a form directly assimilable by the bloodstream. It takes the nutrients processed by spleen and liver and mixes them directly with the blood.

SADDHAK PITTA is located in the heart and is responsible for courage and determination. "Courage" is the result of change in the glucose content of the blood, and "determination" the product of a proper mixture of oxygen in the bloodstream. This *pitta* maintains the balance of both glucose and oxygen.

ALLOCHAK PITTA can be found in the eyes, where it works to aid the vision. *Allochak* balances heat in the eye tissues and muscles and is responsible for regulating light input. When disturbed, diseases of the eyes result.

BHRAJAK PITTA is the most important of the biles, for it provides the *ojas* to the skin and all internal organs. *Ojas* is the viscous fluid responsible for maintaining the glow of health and vitality found on the faces of children and healthy adults. This is the bile which digests the oils which are massaged onto the body, and interacts with the electromagnetic field of the Earth. At the time any problem comes to the system, *bhrajak* is withdrawn, and with it the flow of the *ojas* leaves, as the vital fluid is called in to preserve the afflicted region.

LYMPH: KAPHA is a white, smooth, cold, sticky, sweet fluid which can be found throughout the body. *Tamasic* in nature, it is responsible for moistening and lubricating the system, aids in digestion and helps keep the body clean and pure. It assumes an acidic taste when digested.

As with *vayu* and *pitta, kapha* is one in nature but broken down into five classifications based on location and nature:

KLEYDAN KAPH can be found in the stomach, where it gives added moisture to the freshly chewed food and thus helps separate the bulk into individual particles. By its action the stomach is able to churn and thus hasten the digestive process.

AVLUMBUN KAPH can be found in the heart, where it separates the most powerful nutrients from the blood's chemical soup to provide energy to the heart. It is also found in the head, and in the joints of the bones (where it helps in articulation). This fluid aids in the growth of the bone marrow, which in turn produces the disease-fighting white corpuscles which mix into the bloodstream after first passing through the lymphatic system.

RUSSUN KAPH lives in the throat. Its job is to take the potent nutrients isolated by *avlumbun,* reintroducing the now more powerful chemicals (because they have been isolated for quick metabolism) back into the bloodstream for distribution throughout the system.

SNEHAN KAPH is located in the head, and it is this lymphatic fluid which keeps the delicate tissues of the head moist and well-lubricated. Preventing dryness and dehydration, especially that caused by the constant drying effect of the flow of air through the nostrils, is its primary job. *Snehan* circulates glucose in a high-protein base (mixed with other important chemicals) to the brain. This lymph flows continuously to keep all passages in the head clean and clear from obstruction. *Snehan* is also the carrier of positive and negative ions which are crucial in proper function of the sense organs. This lymph provides the organism with the sense of satisfaction and imparts smoothness to the skin.

SCHLESMA KAPH has also been called phlagellum, and provides binding for the joints.

Each major organ and system has its own lymphatic system, but in type and action the lymph fits well into this classical system of understanding.

Vayu, pitta and *kapha* — wind, bile and mucous — These things are responsible for the play of the body as *sattva, rajas* and *tamas* are responsible for the play of all creation. And as *sattva* and *tamas* are powerless to do anything without the help of *rajas,* so too do *pitta* and *kapha* depend on *vayu* to move them to their required places throughout the body. It is *vayu* which is the key to the whole game. More diseases are caused by *vayu* than by *pitta* and *kapha* combined — and diseases of the lymphatic and bile systems are communicated to other sites in the body by air's circulatory action.

Of all the *vayus, prana vayu* is the key — for without *prana* the other four airs could not work, and without the action of the five airs, death comes instantaneously. It is for this reason that the practice of breath control exercises such as *pranayama* (incorporated in the MEDITATION chapter) are the key to health and well-being. Control of the *prana* automatically gives control of the other four airs. And control of the airs of the body controls the flow and regulation of lymph and bile.

Tridoshas and Individual Systems

No two individuals are exactly alike in physical makeup. Yet this does not mean that each person is a totally unique system. Each individual is like other individuals in many respects, and that group of similar-but-not-identical individuals comprises a "class".

Body chemistry varies according to the dominance of the *tridoshas*. A man dominated by an excess of air behaves, looks and thinks differently than a man dominated by an excess of bile. Physical structure, personality and thought mode all depend on the chemicals and electrolytes present in the system.

The state of body chemistry in the individual is not constant, but varies according to place, climate, diet and a score of other factors. One element may be dominant one day, and another the next. But there is between this daily ebb and flow a larger pattern, the basic chemical blueprint on which the organism has been constructed. This is the genetic code which dictates the definitions of the individual organism.

Seen in this light, there are classes of men who are clearly dominated by the air element; others dominated by bile; others by lymph; still others by air and bile; others by air and lymph; still others by lymph and bile; and a seventh in whom the elements appear in equal measure and balance.

These seven basic classes form the octave of human body chemistry. And of the seven, the basic three classes are *vayu*-dominated, *pitta*-dominated and *kapha*-dominated. This triad corresponds rather closely to the ectomorph-mesomorph-endomorph system of physiological classification (somatotypes) worked out by the American psychologist, William Shelton, and with the extrovert-centrovert-introvert system of psychological classification evolved by the Swiss psychotherapist, Carl Gustav Jung.

The *VAYU*-DOMINATED INDIVIDUAL corresponds to the ectomorph and extrovert. He sleeps little, remains awake most of the time, walks fast and talks too much. His hair is thin, sparse and brittle; his body dry. He has a restless mind, his feelings roaming from place to place almost continuously. He can be cruel, criminal and destructive and suffers from unstable intellect. He does not form fast friendships, and has a weak memory. The air-temperament gives a dislike of cold and cold items. The gestures of such a person are apt to be choppy and quick, and many of the sentences he speaks will be left incomplete as his mind leaves one train of thought and abruptly switches to another. His walk has a lilt, a jaunty quality, reflecting a love of sexual and sensual enjoyments (tastes, smells, singing, dancing, hunting and violence). He is especially fond of sweet, sour, hot and pungent tastes, and produces sound as he drinks water. He eats too much, however. Though strongly built, he is weak in reality and will live a relatively short lifespan. He stammers when he talks.

A master of his sense organs, he is loved by women (but will father few offspring). In dreams he dwells on the mountains, in the trees and in the air — and is sure to have dreams of flying without mechanical aids. His hair will have split ends, and are slightly grayish in colour. The eyes are round and devoid of beauty, being grayish and dry in appearance. When he sleeps, his eyes are ajar like those of a cadaver. The body of this physical type is tall and thin, with the knees especially "knobby" and gnarled. The sounds he makes, his body shape, constitution and mannerisms are like those of a dog, jackal, camel, coyote, rat and owl.

The *PITTA*-DOMINATED INDIVIDUAL corresponds to the mesomorph and the centrovert. The hairs of this type become white at a very early age. Very angry in disposition, he sweats profusely. Learned, brave and proud, he loves flowers and aromatic scents. A man of very good character, his outlook is holy. He earns through means of his own devising and survives by his own efforts. Kind and courageous, he saves even his own worst enemies (who fear him). His eyes are red, and his attachment to the opposite sex minimal. He does not follow the prevalent or current religion and may be opposed to institutionalized religion entirely. He loves sweet, bitter and astringent tastes and is especially fond of cold drinks. He eats a great deal.

The body of the bile-dominated native also smells of his element, and this bile scent becomes especially strong when his anger is roused. Very jealous in nature, he goes to the bathroom frequently. His colour is fair and his body temperature hot. Hands, face and feet are ruddy, and there is less body hair (all hair will be lighter in colour, often yellowish). Loose of joints and muscles, he has less virility and less sexual desire. His eyes immediately get red when angered, intoxicated or exposed to sunlight.

The lifespan of the *pitta*-dominated native is average in length. He dislikes living or visiting places where there are quarrels, and avoids disturbances.

In dreams he sees fire, stars, falling stars, sun, moon, lightning, poisonous plants, and shining objects. His physique, nature and manners may be compared to those of a tiger, bear, wolf or monkey.

The *KAPHA*-DOMINATED INDIVIDUAL has a forgiving disposition and a great deal of virility. His body is well constructed with ample (even excess) fat. His mind is stable and steady, and his nature is sober. His face is moonlike, and his joints well-built, strong, smooth and deep. The body colour of such a person is like brass, gold or a lotus flower. The hands will be long, and the chest strong and broad. Attractive, he has a broad forehead and a tender body with strong, dark, dense and thick hair. The colour of the eyes where the lids meet will be red and smooth. This is a person who is not disturbed by hunger, thirst, pain, disturbance and noise. Wise and fond of order and arrangement, he is a man who honours his own word. He keeps enmity for his enemies for a long time and will seek out secret and devious ways to avenge himself. Yet he follows the principles and practices of right living, and does not speak harsh language. He has a great love of sexual enjoyment.

The sound of the *kapha*-dominated individual is like the ocean, or conch-shell when blown. He will have many sons and subordinates. Industrious and humble, he is slow to anger and takes a great deal of time to complete his work (because he spends much time in thought and fantasy). Sweet-spoken, forgiving and serious in outlook, he is basically a simple person though also very learned. He tries to keep his contacts stable and of long duration. He loves bitter, astringent, sharp and dry tasting foods. He sleeps a great deal.

The dreams of such a person are filled with rivers, ponds, oceans, lakes, lotus and water birds. In temperament, habits and physique he has the traits of elephant, horse, lion, cow and bull.

The Establishment of Chemical Nature

What is it that determines the basic nature of an individual? Body chemistry is created by a man's genes, and the genes are the biological links between parents and children. So the individual body pattern is established by the fusion of genes from the father's sperm cell and the mother's ovum.

Yet the sperm cells discharged by the father are many in number, while the ovum is but one. The sperm cells contain literally millions of genetic permutations, yet of these only one can meet and fuse with the ovum.

Each sperm cell has a slightly different chemical charge, and most sperm cells die before ever reaching near the ovum. Only one cell at any given time has the power to meet with and fertilize the ovum.

Why one cell of millions reaches the goal can be attributed to mere chance — or it can be attributed to a logical and scientific sequence of events.

The mucous lining the organs of the mother varies in chemical composition according to the nature of the chemical present in the mother's system. The chemical soup which coats the innerwalls of the passage leading to the womb is produced by the lymphatic system, and the lymphatic fluids vary subtly in composition each day, from moment to moment, according to the chemicals fed into them by the tissues and glands.

The chemical ocean in which the sperm cell must swim has specific properties, and it is these ever-changing properties which attract or repel specific sperm cells, according to the chemicals present in the genetic material stored by the sperm. Not all sperm cells can reach the ovum because, for them, the passage through the generative organs is inhibited by the presence of chemicals not in harmony with those they are carrying. Only that cell which is in complete harmony with the chemical system of the mother can reach and fertilize the ovum.

It is for this reason that Indian medical texts state that the condition of the mother is 80% the determiner of the nature of the child.

Five factors are listed as determining the body chemistry of the future child. First is the body chemistry of the father at the time of intercourse, which determines what chemicals will be present in the sperm cells. Second is the nature of the genetic chemicals in the ovum. Third is the food taken by the couple in the previous 36 hours — which will go to make up the chemicals in the nutrient fluids. Fourth is the emotional responses of the mother, which set the hormonal content of her lymphatic system (gestures, postures and sounds). Fifth is the general condition of the womb itself.

If the air is the dominant *dosha* in a woman's body, and in her mate's as well; and if the food they have taken in air-dominated; and if her emotional responses are "airy" in nature; and lastly, if her womb is at that moment dominated by *vayu* — if all five of these factors are dominated by *vayu*, then the child born of such congress will be *vayu*-dominated. If all five are *pitta*-dominated, then the child too will be dominated by *pitta*; likewise for *kapha*. Variations within this pattern will produce the other four combinations of *vayu-pitta, vayu-kapha, kapha-pitta* and "balanced".

Detecting Imbalances

In addition to one's basic hereditary and environmental predisposition, the proportions of the *doshas* will vary from day to day according to changes in individual activity, diet and psychological conditions. Each *dosha* produces specific effects as it increases or decreases in the system. A knowledge of these effects is necessary to enable one to take the necessary remedial action.

Disturbed vayu is characterized by excessive thirst, shaking and dryness, roughness, redness of skin, pain, hiccough, asthma, cough; ailments of ears, nose and throat; circulatory troubles, urinary ailments, constipation, etc. If *vayu* is increasing, it creates roughness of voice, emaciation, a desire for heat, throbbing sensations, insomnia, darkened complexion, weakness and constipation. If decreasing, uneasiness, languor and unconsciousness are produced.

Disturbed pitta creates burning sensations, excessive heat, perspiration, acidity, thirst, acne, irritability, redness of the eyes, putrid smells, decomposition, languor, hysteria, indigestion, hyperacidity, sensations of heat in the chest and stomach, expulsion of blood from body openings, lack of imagination, stupor, defective vision, skin deseases (including pigmentation changes) and apoplexy. If *pitta* is increasing, it produces burning sensations, a preference for cold and cooling foods, yellow eyes and complexion, yellow stool and urine, insomnia, fainting and diminished function of sense organs. If decreasing, *pitta* produces dull complexion and diminished body heat.

Disturbed kapha produces heaviness, drowsiness, numbness, pallor, itching, nausea, anorexia, dyspepsia, loss of memory, vitiation of sense, white urine and stool, heaviness and rigidity in the joints and feeling of old age. Often a sweet taste in the mouth is experienced. Increasing *kapha* produces heaviness of the limbs, cold sensations, drowsiness, excessive sleep, looseness of joints and a pallid complexion. Decreasing *kapha* produces dryness, internal burning sensations, feelings of emptiness in the stomach and lower tract, looseness of joints (due to dryness), thirst, weakness and insomnia

The Doshas and Taste

To maintain a proper balance in body chemistry, one should be aware of the play of elements within his own system. Armed with this knowledge he can then orchestrate the rhythm of his body and mind by addhng or subtracting elements from his diet as necessary.

Different foods, according to their particular properties, stimulate or subdue the quantity and action of each of the three *doshas*.

How does one determine which elements are most prevalent in his diet? It is not chemical analysis, but taste, which provides the key. Each element has a characteristic taste, and with an understanding of taste each *dosha* can be dealt with individually.

Rasa, literally "taste", provides the key to self-regulation by diet. *Rasas* are divided into six basic categories, each with a specific effect on body chemistry. The six tastes are sweet, sour, pungent, bitter, salty and astringent. Each is the product of the combination of two elements (*tattwas*):

1. *Madhura Rasa*, the sweet taste, results from the combination of water and earth. Sugar or honey are the purest examples of this *rasa*.
2. *Amla Rasa*, the sour taste, arises from the admixture of water and fire. Lemon, vinegar and yogurt are good examples.
3. *Katu Rasa*, the pungent taste, is formed by air and

fire. Chili peppers and spicy pickles are representative.

4. *Tikta Rasa,* the bitter taste, is produced by the blending of air and *akash.* Bitter melon and quinine are instances of this *rasa.*

5. *Lavana Rasa,* the salty taste, results from the merging of earth and fire. Plain table salt is a good example.

6. *Kshaya Rasa,* the astringent taste, is produced by air and earth. Alum is representative.

These six combinations are directly responsible for the operation and balance of the three *doshas. Vayu* is stimulated by astringent, bitter and pungent tastes; subdued by sweet, sour and salty. *Pitta* is stimulated by bitter, sour and salty; subdued by sweet, astringent and pungent tastes. *Kapha* is stimulated by sweet, sour and salty tastes; subdued by bitter, pungent, and astringent.

Doshas and Diet

By careful observation of the effect of different items of diet, one can gradually begin to formulate a list of basic staples suited to his individual constitution.

In order to acquire an understanding of the nature of specific food items, the founders of *Ayurveda* subsisted on nothing but a single item for periods of 14 days and longer. From their observations have come scores of volumes to which additions are still being made. The discovery of the Americas brought whole new varieties of food previously unknown; potatoes, tomatoes, corn and a score of others. Each of these newcomers was given the same thorough testing in the laboratory of the body.

The most easily observed of qualities is the effect of foods on the *doshas.* Foods accordingly are classified by their *dosha* properties.

Vayu foods: Foods containing *vayu* and little or no *pitta* or *kapha* strengthen the nervous system, but weaken the mucous and circulatory system.

Pitta foods: strengthen circulation, but weaken the mucosal and nervous systems.

Kapha foods: strengthen the mucous system, weakening nerves and circulation.

Vayu-pitta foods: strengthen nerves and circulation at the expense of the mucous system.

Vayu-kapha foods: strengthen nerves and mucous, weaken circulation and increase the concentration of heat.

Pitta-kapha foods: Extremely unusual, they promote circulation and lubrication, weakening the nerves.

Vayu-pitta-kapha foods: promote proper function of all bodily systems.

A diet containing all three elements in the proper proportion is most beneficial for the human system. But one must learn for himself what proportions are best suited for his own system.

Foods containing all three elements number four: fresh, whole milk, fresh cream, black pepper and fish. Fish is not desirable for the reasons discussed in the section on vegetarianism. The milk and cream must be of the same day's milking, otherwise the *vayu* and *pitta* properties will be lost, leaving only *kapha* (the only element remaining in store-purchased milk). Whole milk or cream should be taken only after heating to just below the boiling point.

Black peppers are the most powerful of all tonics, and their medicinal value will be discussed in the Home Remedies chapter. Following is an alphabetical listing of some common foods with their properties in terms of the *tridoshas*:

Avocado — *kapha*

Banana — *vayu-pitta*

Beets — *vayu-kapha*

Broccoli — *vayu*

Cabbage — *kapha*

Carrots — *vayu-kapha*

Cauliflower — *kapha*

Celery — *pitta*

Chestnuts — *vayu-kapha*

Chocolate — *pitta*

Coffee — *pitta*

Corn — *vayu-kapha*

Cornflakes and meal — *vayu*

Cream — *vayu-pitta-kapha*

Cream cheese — *vayu-kapha*

Curds — *pitta*

Dates — *vayu-kapha*

Endive — *pitta-kapha*

Escarol — *kapha*

Grapefruit — *kapha*

Grapes — *vayu-kapha*

Greens — *kapha*

Honey — *kapha*

Kelp — *kapha*

Kolrabi — *kapha*

Lemon — *vayu*

Lettuce — *kapha*

Milk (fresh whole)
 —*vayu-pitta-kapha*

Milk (bottled) — *kapha*

Mint — *pitta*

Mushrooms — *kapha*

Oatmeal — *vayu-kapha*

Olives (ripe) — *vayu-kapha*

Onions — *pitta*

Parsley — *vayu*

Parsnips — *pitta*

Peanuts — *pitta*

Pears — *kapha*

Peas — *pitta*

Persimmons — *kapha*

Pickles (sour and hot) — *pitta*

Potatoes — *pitta*

Pulses — *pitta* .

Rice — *kapha*

Salt — *vayu*

Soyabeans — *pitta*

Spinach — *kapha*

Squash — *vayu*

Sugar (raw) — *pitta*

Sugar (refined) — *vayu-pitta*

Sunflower seeds — *pitta*

Swiss chard — *kapha*

Tea — *vayu*

Tomatoes — *kapha*

Turnips — *kapha*

Vinegar — *pitta*

Walnuts — *pitta*

Wheat — *pitta*

Foods and Systemic Action

Both foods and medication are also classed according to their action on the system as a whole. This is referred to as *veerya* or power, the two main groupings of which are hot and cold — *ushna* and *shita*. *Ushna* has the properties of combustion, digestion, vomiting, purging, destroying *vayu* and *kapha*, increasing *pitta*, imparting a feeling of lightness to the body and destroying semen. The cold power, *shita*, creates steadiness, nourishment increases *vayu* and *kapha*, increases heaviness, imparts strength and nourishment, and aids in the build-up of body fluids.

Foods are also classified on the basis of their interaction with the digestive system itself. This process of chemical interaction creates specific effects, called *vipakas*. Light foods (*laghu vipaka*) cause constipation, promote gas and destroy *kapha*. Heavy foods (*guru vipaka*) destroy *vayu* and *pitta*, promote *kapha*, aid in clearing urine and stool from the system. Sour, bitter and pungent-tasting foods are light, while salt, astringent and sweet foods are heavy.

Taste, *doshas,* chemical effect and post-digestive action form the basis of dietary understanding in the *Ayurvedic* system. With a proper understanding of these principles, anyone can formulate a diet which will establish and maintain health and well-being.

Food and the Gunas

As the three *gunas* can be found in human physiology, so too can they be found in the food which constitutes the human diet.

Some food is more *sattvic* in nature: it produces a high yield of directly useable energy with the least possible expenditure of digestive effort. Food of this nature is suitable as the basic dietary staple of those living quiet, contemplative existences.

Some food is more *rajasic* in nature. These items of diet produce a great deal of activity in the human system with a moderate amount of digestive effort. A diet of *rajasic* staples is suitable for someone living in the world who does not need to expend a great deal of physical power.

Some food is more *tamasic* in nature: while harder to digest, it produces a great amount of potential heat energy which can be stored by the system. Food of this type is best suited for those who must do a great deal of hard physical labour.

How to tell which item of food is which? While the nature of energy varies from food to food, it is none-theless possible to group food into three basic types according to the manner in which it is grown.

Tamasic foods are those which grow on or under the ground. Root crops, peanuts and those parts of a plant which touch the surface of the earth are *tamasic* in nature. Examples include potatoes, yams, peanuts, beets and rutabagas.

Tamasic foods are strong and dense and provide the staple and support for a plant. They are those parts of the plant most directly bound by gravity, and contain the heaviest, most *tamasic* energy.

The *rajasic* parts of plants are those parts which have to do with the manufacture and conveyance and nutri-ments. Included in this category are leaves, stems and branches. It is these parts of the plant which provide the basic nutritional energy which the plant needs to live. They are most active (*rajasic*) parts of the plant, and it is by their action that moisture is drawn up from the roots.

It is the *rajasic* parts of the plant which preserve the day-to-day well-being of the plant.

The *sattvic* parts of the plant are those which contain the essence of the plant. Only the seeds themselves fit into this category, for it is the seed which contains the whole plant in microcosmic form.

The ultimate purpose of life is to reproduce, each according to its own kind. The seeds contain the purest and most subtle form of energy produced by the plant, and are thus the most *sattvic* part.

Fruits, however, are *rajasic* in nature. Seeds are contained within a fruit, but the bulk of the fruit is consumed by food reservers for the seed (which serve to attract animals which will carry the seeds as well). While the seeds themselves are *sattvic* in nature, the mass of the fruit itself is *rajasic* (and the skin itself may be *tamasic,* if thick and moisture proof). Thus a pumpkin seed is *sattvic*, the pulp *rajasic* and the skin *tamasic*. The seed reproduces the plant, and is its essence. The pulp nourishes and preserves the seed, and is its activity. The skin provides stability and inertness.

By this same token, both wheat and rice are primarily *rajasic*, for the bulk of the kernel is nutriment for the small germ, which is the real *sattvic* part (the seed).

These are basic rules, which can generally be used to determine the nature of most food items. It should always be remembered that canned and preserved foods are never *sattvic*, and may be *rajasic* at best (though all canned foods are *tamasic*).

It is also a rule of thumb that *tamasic* foods generate the most gas in digestion; *sattvic* foods the least. It is also true that some foods change in nature according to their manner of preparation (most raw nuts are *tamasic* to the system because they are impossible to digest, becoming *sattvic* when allowed to germinate by standing overnight in water, then being ground into an easily digested paste).

Nine

Diet : Specific Foods

Some foods are good at one time of day, but not another. Some foods are the best guarantors of health in one season, yet the causes of disease a few months later. Similarly, some foods which do well alone become poison in combination. The following pages illustrate these points, as well as provide an Indian perspective of some of the more common staples of diet.

Cold Weather Foods

People in cold climates eat meat because it provides an abundance of raw energy to help maintain body heat, but what foods will provide the necessary heat for vegetarians in these climates? Fortunately, meat is not the only source of heat. There are a great variety of vegetarian staples which can more than compensate for lower temperatures.

Black pepper, red pepper, onions and especially garlic are four spices which should be used in cold weather cooking.

Almonds, cashews, walnuts and pistachios — always roasted first — make good

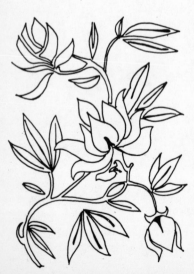

supplements to the diet, as do raisin. Dishes containing potatoes, tomatoes, turnips, carrots, onion, spinach, greens, squash, and cooked cucumbers provide energy which will add heat to the system, as will sweet peas.

Cracked wheat, oat and tapioca cereals make good breakfast foods, especially prepared with freshly roasted nuts and raisins. Dates and figs are good as well.

As a general rule, dairy products and citrus fruits should be avoided because they are sour foods and produce cold in the system. The only permissible dairy product is cheese. Bananas are good among the fruits, and some papaya, mango and pomegranate may be taken. The honey and black pepper mixture described in the section on medicines should be taken first thing each morning. Following this a small garlic clove can be swallowed with lukewarm water.

A tea made with a teaspoon or more of fenugreek seeds, a teaspoon of chopped ginger, seven black peppercorns and black tea is an instant heat-producer.

Hot Weather Foods

As there are special foods for winter, so too there are items of diet which enable one to synchronize with the temperature and pressure changes heralded by the onset of summer.

Hot weather dehumidifies the system causing the blood to thicken. Hence one should take foods with a high moisture content in a diet well-laced with frequent breaks for any one of a number of pleasing and healthful beverages.

Summer also triggers a change in the body's fat content. The system naturally accumulates stored calories in the form of fat during the winter months as a protection against the cold. With the start of summer the system automatically consumes the stored fat, which would otherwise burden the body chemistry during the hot summer months. This process of combustion of stored fat releases a great deal of heat into the system, which produces additional dehydration.

While the burning of stored fat increases the glucose content of the bloodstream, the combination of summer heat and internal heat further dries the system, producing a pronounced thickening of the blood. The vital fluid becomes dense and sluggish, and less glucose and other nutrients reach the brain because the heart pumps less blood with the same amount of effort required to pump more of the thinner blood of winter.

For this reason, one should be especially careful to augment his diet at the start of summer with one or more gallons of liquid intake, balanced with added natural sugars.

Canteloupe, berries of all kinds, peaches, pears, apricots, plums, watermelon, pineapple, grapes, oranges and other fresh and easily digestible fruit make excellent items of diet for the summer. Fruits are *sattvic* foods (though watermelon and canteloupe are *tamasic*), and provide most of the nutriments needed for life. One who eats seasonally fresh locally grown fruit during the summer need not eat other items of diet. This may be done as a fasting discipline.

All leafy green vegetables are excellent and provide the body with natural salts lost in perspiration. Mustard greens, spinach, collard, turnip tops, beet tops and other "greens" are especially good. Watercress is of great value, either raw in salads or cooked as a vegetable.

Rutabagas, turnips, radish, pumpkins, all types of squash (especially zucchini) and cucumbers may form the basic dietary staples, along with greens and fruits. Cucumbers are especially good — raw with lemon juice and salt sprinkled on top, or cooked. Yogurt too is excellent. Because the heat naturally present in beans disappears when the beans have germinated, sprouts are also a good food for summer time.

Mint is an excellent food to cool the system, and may be used as a garnish (either chopped fresh or dry leaves sprinkled directly on food), made into tea or ground into a paste with water and used as a chutney (add salt and a few pomegranate seeds for best flavour).

Cumin is the spice for summer use, and should be used whenever possible. Turmeric and coriander should be used as frequently as possible in winter — but *not* in summer. Other spices which should be avoided during the hot season are cloves, cardamom, garlic, onion and cinnamon. Garlic and ginger may be used — but only in small quantities and for medicinal purposes (as both kill gas).

Summer Beverages

Because water is the fuel of fire, the use of as much liquid as possible safeguards the system during the firey summer months. One who keeps his system well flushed with water and fresh beverages minimizes the dehumidifying effects of summer heat and insures good health for the duration of the season.

There are many pleasant-tasting beverages which provide both liquid and nutritional value to protect against the adverse effects of the season.

The most basic drink is cold water and honey — one which both thins the blood and provides an immediate boost in glucose content to the brain. Lemon juice in cold water with either honey or raw sugar to taste also provides a lift for both the bloodstream and the digestive tract. Fruit juices of all kinds, freshly squeezed from fresh fruits, are always good in summer — though all sour drinks and foods should be taken only during sunlight hours, never at night.

For a special treat, one can make a drink called *shikunji*. Make a lemonade using mineral water, lemon juice and raw sugar or honey, adding a pinch of salt, fresh mint and a dash of either cinnamon or freshly ground black pepper. This delightful mix compensates for all the seasonal adversities — the glucose of the sweetener and the salt together righting the balance of blood and brain chemistry.

To make another pleasant and healthful drink, begin by soaking a package of dried tamarind overnight in water. When the fruit has become soft, grind it into a paste with water (a blender may be used), then filter through a cheesecloth. Take the filtered juice and add water to make the consistency of apple juice. Now add a pinch of salt, a sprig of mint, a few raisins and either raw sugar or honey to taste. A pinch of cinnamon may be added if desired. For a special treat, add a pinch of freshly powdered cumin. This drink is of great benefit on especially hot days — for the "Dog Days" and doldrums.

A Special Drink

This next drink is a special summertime treat which everyone will enjoy. Begin with the following ingredients:

- ½ cup shelled canteloupe seeds
- ½ cup shelled pumpkin seeds
- 2 tablespoons white poppy seeds
- 1 tablespoon anise seed
- 1 handful of dried wild rose petals
  (available at many health food stores and Mexican food shops)
- ½ cup raw milk
- 7 black peppercorns
- Raw sugar or honey

Soak all seeds but the peppercorns overnight (at least six hours). Grind the seeds and petals into a paste, using sufficient water, either in a blender or a mortar and pestle. Now strain the paste through a cheesecloth to remove potentially harmful particles and add the raw milk to the strained liquid. Add enough water to bring the mixture to the consistency of whole milk, then add sugar or honey to taste. A few drops of rosewater may be added.

This drink is both refreshing and invigorating, providing the body with natural sugars, vitamin C and other vitamins, and a large amount of protein which is of great value to the system.

Summer and Yogurt

Because of its cooling nature, its wealth of B-complex vitamins and its general tonic effect on the system yogurt should be made a staple item of the summer diet. Made in the home from fresh, whole milk, yogurt provides most of the nutrients required by the human system. Yogurt may be served by itself or used as the base for fruit salads. There are several delightful drinks made from this relatively complete food.

The yogurt which provides the best nutritional qualities and finest energy is yogurt which has been made fresh in the home out of whole, raw milk. Yogurt made at home from pasteurized milk is, however, still preferable to the yogurt generally found in stores (which is old and often made from skim milk and powdered milk products).

To make fresh yogurt, simply boil a half-gallon of milk in a large saucepan. Once the milk has boiled, remove the pan from the heat, cover with a cheesecloth or strainer (to keep out impurities) and allow to cool almost to room temperature. Once the yogurt has cooled, add ¼ cup of commercial yogurt or yogurt culture to start the yeast in the cooled milk.

Take the milk to which the culture has been added, cover and keep in a warm (not hot) place. One may use a warming tray, an oven set on "warm" with the door left well ajar, or any oven in which a hundred-watt lightbulb is burning. The yogurt will "set" in about eight hours.

Glass is the best medium for preparing yogurt, though stainless steel is also good. Under no circumstances should yogurt be made in aluminium containers, for yogurt is acidic in nature and will break down the aluminium into potentially poisonous compounds. As a general rule, aluminium cookware should be avoided for this reason — all acidic foods break down aluminium.

After the yogurt has set, remove from warmth and keep in the refrigerator at least one full day. This is to stop the action of the yeast on the milk before the milk is completely consumed. Yogurt should always be cooled at least one day before serving, or its taste and texture will not be good.

One of the best summer drinks is *lassi*, prepared from yogurt.

To make *lassi*, churn fresh, cooled yogurt with an egg-beater until it has become well blended. A foam will rise to the top containing small particles of butter. Stop churning when the foam becomes thick and without butter. Now add water to make the drink the consistency of fresh milk, using rosewater and sugar or honey to taste. *Lassi* is cooling, refreshing — and provides the system with a healthy measure of B-12 and other yeast-generated vitamins.

Lassi may also be made directly from raw milk, sugar, water and rosewater when yogurt is not available, or as a variation.

Morning Foods

Foods should be eaten according to the time of day. How one begins the day is critical. Morning is the *sattvic* time of day, from ninety minutes before sunrise to mid-day, thus only *sattvic* food should be taken during this time.

Most cereals are acceptable. Oats and wheat are especially good, though they should only be taken in small quantities. Seeds and nuts are good, though they should always be roasted beforehand. Exceptions are the pignola (pine nut) and the almond, neither of which needs roasting.

Three to five pignolas may be eaten without any preparation. Only one or two almonds should be taken after being soaked overnight in cool water. Before eating, peel and grind the almond into a fine paste on a slightly rough stone. Use a few drops of water as needed and grind in a clockwise direction.

Pine nuts are the best of all nuts, the only seed which can be taken whole and raw. They are a great food and Hindus believe they cure a broad variety of diseases.

Citrus fruits, which are a *rajasic* food, should never be taken in the morning. *Rajasic* foods taken at a *sattvic* time create a state of hypersensitivity and anger in those susceptible.

Sattvic fruits which can be taken are: grapes, guavas, bananas, pears, raisins, and the seed of canteloupe and watermelon — but not the fruit which is *tamasic* (it grows on the ground). Coconut is an excellent *sattvic* food. The milk of coconut is both *sattvic* and alkaline and when taken regularly (one-third of the juice of a medium coconut) kills stomach acidity and anger. Taken as the only morning intake for 40 days, it can cure all stomach problems and abate chronic anger. Both the meat and milk of coconut are good for *prana*.

Afternoon Foods

In the afternoon one needs juices and foods with a greater liquid content. From the time of the thinning of the blood at ten minutes before dawn, the blood slowly and gradually loses power. From shortly before noon to mid-afternoon, the system is at the peak of activity, consuming energy at a rapid pace to insure that daily routine is completed. By late afternoon the system is fully exhausted.

In the afternoon then, the system needs food which provides energy with the minimum amount of effort. This is therefore the customary time for tea and other stimulants. To compensate for the toxins of caffeine and theaine, one should only take coffee and tea with roasted nuts in the winter; cucumber, canteloupe and pumpkin seed in summer.

Fruit juices are good in the afternoon during summer, as are fresh fruits. One should eat only lightly if activity remains to be completed, for actions taken when the stomach is full create an imbalance in the body gases which can lead to many different types of disease.

Yogurt and fruit make a good combination — though neither yogurt nor fruit should be taken within an hour of tea. Also bananas and yogurt should not be mixed.

Evening Foods

By evening, the body's energy has been largely expended, and what remains is largely centred in the head (it is this which makes the night the time for talking and joking). Because so little energy remains, the food taken in the evening hours should be both light and easily digested.

After sunset the ionic charge of the atmosphere drops, and the later one eats, the more likely the food is to be improperly digested.

Citrus foods should be avoided at night because the vitamin D and citric acid stimulate the production of urine, and the need for urination can disturb an otherwise sound sleep. This is true for all acidic foods, as acid stimulates urination, as well as thinning the semen.

While nuts and seed are good for breakfast, soups, boiled vegetables, yeast bread, beans and greens are excellent in the evening. Both yogurt and rice, however, should be avoided. Root foods (potatoes, beets, etc.) should not be taken at night, as they require a great deal of digestive effort.

Recently, dietary studies have determined that carbohydrates increase activity and circulation in the brain, while animal proteins dull the brain (though the protein found in almond paste, cashews and other freshly roasted or pasted nuts is highly refined and not dulling). Thus one should avoid high-protein foods in the evening, and nuts are best taken only in the morning.

Fried foods should be avoided at night, and no oils used in preparing the evening meal. Fewer spices should be used in cooking at night — and bachelors should avoid all hot and spicy food after dark.

The right foods taken in the evening insure a clean and prompt bowel movement the next morning. Papaya is especially good at night. If one boils either dates or raisins in milk just before retiring, the morning movement will be clean and prompt. Warm milk is also relaxing to the system and gives good sleep — and by itself helps give clean bowels (although bachelors should avoid raw milk at night).

As a general rule, cereal is good for the morning, fruits and juices for the afternoon, and boiled vegetables and pulpy foods in the evening.

Wheat

"Man cannot live by bread alone", goes the old adage. But fresh whole-wheat bread, a few well-cooked vegetables and a glass of buttermilk, all given a light dash of black pepper, can provide a lifetime of health for any man.

Wheat has justly been called the monarch of foods. No other dietary staple, save fresh yogurt buttermilk, provides such greatly concentrated nourishment for all seven bodily tissues (bone, marrow, muscles, nerves, skin, semen, and blood). And of all grains and cereals, wheat is the most readily digested by the human system because of its capacity to absorb water — which in turn conducts heat uniformly throughout the grain.

Wheat is the only food which should *not* be taken fresh. Kernels freshly plucked from the stalk contain a greater quantity of solar energy than the human system can adequately handle. Therefore no wheat should be taken which has not been aged for at least four months — or soaked overnight in water and allowed to sun-dry for three days. So great is the solar energy concentrated in wheat that granaries storing vast quantities of this nutritious grain must be thoroughly and continuously ventilated — or spontaneous combustion can generate fire, even explosions in freshly-ground flour.

Stored and soaked wheat remains fertile, but the excessive solar energy is discharged into the atmosphere instead of the stomach.

In whatever form it is taken, wheat should always be thoroughly browned first. Breads should always be toasted, or — and this is preferable — thin tortilla-like breads should be prepared fresh at each meal and either fried dry or on a lightly oiled pan on medium-high heat, or french fried. Wheat cereals should also be browned in a dry, unoiled pan on medium-high heat before the addition of water. Cracked wheat cereal prepared in this fashion provides on excellent breakfast food.

Wheat is sweet in taste, cold in power and heavy in post-digestive action. Rich in vitamins, minerals, proteins, carbohydrates and a score of other nutrients, it may be taken with any meal on any occasion. The gluten content in wheat provides physical endurance and sexual stamina —which is why celibates should eat less wheat products than married individuals unless engaged in hard physical labour.

Whole wheat flour is always preferable to the "en-riched" white pastes, and fresh bread always better than store-bought.

Rice

Second only to wheat in nourishment and utility among the grains is rice. There is one major difference between rice and wheat, however — rice creates gas in the system, regardless of how it is cooked. For this reason all patients of gastritis or constipation should avoid this food.

The white varieties of rice are preferable to brown rice — the brown varieties are very hard to digest and create far more gastric distress.

All varieties are sweet in taste, cool in action and promote gas, forming scanty and condensed stools.

Rice can be prepared in dozens of ways, from appetizers to desserts. Breads made of rice flour are very popular in Southern India, where rice serves most of the role wheat plays in the rest of the world.

Cloves and shredded coconut may be added to any rice dish to counteract the gastric upset. And because rice is a cold (Moon) food, it should either be avoided in cold climates or prepared with roasted nuts, seeds or peas to provide heat.

Fruits

APRICOTS: The apricot is a favourite food in the North West Himalayas. It has been used there since times immemorial as a main food because it provides a great deal of nourishment.

Apricots are similar in shape to peaches and also have nuts inside them. The nut is sold in the market and oil is extracted from its kernel. This oil is as good as almond oil. Apricots are a rich source of protein, carbohydrate, sodium, calcium, magnesium, phosphorus, sulphur, copper, iron and chlorine. The apricot is also supposed to be an excellent source of vitamin A and dry apricots contain three times more vitamin A than fresh ones.

Apricots taken in large amounts (ranging from six to twelve) by patients with chronic constipation help the evacuation of the bowels. The apricot also helps patients with anaemia because of its rich iron and calcium content and because it is supposed to increase the production of haemoglobin.

Dry apricots must be soaked overnight in water before being eaten, and before soaking they must be properly washed because the water in which they are soaked can be drunk as it will be rich with apricot-juice. Apricots can also be soaked in milk, or boiled with milk. The milk is a powerful drink because this way the apricots are most easily digested.

Soaked apricots can be used in salads, chutneys and saunth in place of tamarindum. For making saunth the compressed pulp of apricots is very good.

BANANA (Sweet and Ripe): The banana is a holy food and is very popular in Prasad (consecrated food). Banana is useful in cases of dysentery, diarrhoea, chronic indigestion and for people suffering from weak digestive fire. As a fruit it is a great tonic and it provides the system with a lot of nutrient materials.

Ripe bananas are popular everywhere. They have different shapes and sizes according where they grow, but the banana with the golden yellow skin and brown spots is one of the best tasting varieties.

According to Ayurvedic texts the banana is a tasty, appetizing fibre and flesh-building fruit and it is thirst-quenching. It is slightly constipating, but if used properly and regularly bananas remove and cure constipation. They also cure diseases caused by wind (*Vayu*), bile (*Pitta*) and mucous (*Kapha*), they increase semen and they increase vitality and virility. Bananas cure all kinds of weaknesses and they help cure diabetes and sper-matorea.

For people who are bony, skinny and thin the banana is an ideal food. Thin people should eat two bananas after food regularly for a few months. This will help them to gain weight without getting fat and it will help them to look more beautiful. For those who urinate often, or who are suffering from diabetes bananas are very good. They will reduce the disease and help them. Because of being sweet the banana increases the amount of semen and thus increases strength, stamina, vitality and virility. For people who have exhausted themselves by over-indulgence in sexual games bananas are very useful, they fill them up and make them strong again.

For dry coughs, hooping cough or any other type of

cough trouble a drink made from bananas is extremely beneficial.

Bananas are slightly constipating if taken in small quantities. One large banana, or two or three small bananas eaten one after the other will however remove constipation. Bananas solidify stools and can be given to children from two months of age on without any problem. Eat bananas if you have teeth, drink them if you don't have teeth. Bananas digest well and easily, but do not eat too little of them. Regularly eating bananas, oranges and apples keeps the system healthy.

It is advisable to eat a banana after food, it helps the digestion. The banana has plenty of calories, vitamins A and C and many mineral salts. It has 75.3% water, it has a number of carbohydrates, little protein, very little fat and it has calcium, phosphorous, iron, thiamine, riboflavin, niacin, magnesium, copper, sulphur and potassium.

Flour can be made from dried bananaflakes. Pancakes made from this flour are very delicious and satisfying. Bananaflour is more nutritive than that of cereals. Ripe bananas with milk, nuts and seeds, or bananas in muesli make a good breakfast. The banana has a high percentage of alkali and helps maintain the alkaline reserve of the body. It is ideal food for gastric ulcers, gastritis and ulcerative colitis.

Recipe for a banana dish: Slice small flakes from about a dozen bananas. Add an equal amount in weight of raw sugar and add water, cover the pot with a lid. Set the pot over a low flame. When the water starts boiling, remove the pot and let it cool. Add a little saffron and one green cardamom per person and serve.

In cases of weak digestive fire bananas can be given with tamarindum and salt. Bananas are a cure for children with dysentery; one banana thoroughly mashed is a good remedy.

Bananas help building bones and are very helpful in jaundice, because of their iron content. They are also good in acute gout and arthritis.

Eating bananas helps the heart and when there is pain in the heart bananas blended with honey can be life-savers. Bananas with honey are an ideal *sattvik* food. To this a pinch of saffron can also be added.

The skin of bananas placed wherever there is muscular pain, or pain resulting from scratching prevents swelling and relieves pain. The banana skin is germproof.

If by chance one eats more than a reasonable amount of bananas and one experiences indigestion, one red cardamom should be taken. Red cardamom dissolves bananas and makes them digestible within a few minutes.

DATES: Dates are hot and dry, they give power to the stomach, cure diseases of wind and mucous and they are slightly constipating. Dates are very useful for those suffering from a cough and dates put on weight. If buttermilk is taken after eating dates it will immediately digest them.

Dates are found in India in two main varieties. One variety is big, sweet and tasty, the other variety is small and not so sweet.

Dates are used as sugar (jaggery or *gur*) and as candies in certain parts of India. They are very rich in food value. Their taste is sweet and that is why they are very satisfying. Dates give strength, stamina, vitality and virility and they increase semen, Those who have exhausted themselves by overindulgence in sex, those who are always depressed and those who feel tired and worn out should eat quite a lot of dates every day for several months. Their sugar is easily digestible and provides enough calories. Dates can be eaten after a meal and if someone wants to increase his strength he should eat about fifteen to twenty dates at one time once a day. This person should also take a minimum of half a litre milk and he should exercise. Within forty days one is physically and mentally strong and rejuvenated.

In cases of injury where lots of blood is lost, if the patient is given dates and milk with a little ghee or cream it will immediately help.

For patients of anaemia and general weakness dates with milk and cream at breakfast is very helpful. For those who feel they are loosing stamina datemilk is a tonic. Those who feel they do not have clear bowel movements in the morning should drink milk boiled with four, five or more dates before going to sleep at night. Dates have a good quantity of vitamins A, B and C and this combination gives the system the power of resistance against viruses and infections. Dates also contain protein, minerals, carbohydrates, calcium, phosphorous, iron, thiamin, niacin, pectin and riboflavin which makes them rejuvenators. Dates can be used in many ways as sweets, vegetables, pickles and sour chutneys.

Dates work as a cleanser and expel mucous, thus they have a medicinal value for ailments of the chest region and for coughs. Dates provides strength to the heart, liver, digestive glands and kidneys. They help in building the nerves in the brain area and they increase appetite. They are tissue builders. In the Medieval Health Handbook dates are described as cold and dry, good for the intestines and dangerous for the throat and chest. They are recommended eaten with honeycomb and are considered a very suitable food for the old and debilitated, for those convalescing and for children. Regular use of dates establishes a colony of friendly bacteria in the intestine.

Dates are potentially alkaline in nature. They keep an alkali balance in the system, are regarded as a health food and are bloodstrengthening.

Rich Arabs eat dates filled with butter. The carbohydrate content of dates helps the digestion of butter. Dates are also supposed to be a holy food. The dateplant and the coconutplant belong to the same genus and both are holy.

FIGS: Figs are a holy food; the same as dates, coconuts and bananas. The fig is a fruit that can be eaten both fresh and dried. It is allowed to ripen on the tree and the ripe fruits which fall down are collected and either eaten or kept for drying. The ripe fig is palatable sweet in taste, it is cold in nature, it aids the digestive process and it helps the system get rid of impurities in the blood. Figs subdue the humours wind and bile. They contain protein, minerals, sodium, potassium, calcium, iron, copper, magnesium, phosphorous, sulphur and chlorine. Figs are always recommended for all chest troubles and for constipation, and also they are for chronic coughs. The syrup of figs is an excellent tonic for infants, increasing their appetite and improving digestion. Fig-syrup also cures muscular rheumatism, seminal disorders, skin troubles, kidney stones, bladder stones, enlargements of the liver and leucorrhoea. It is therefore advisable for women to eat two figs a day. Because of their iron content they are prescribed to patients with anaemia. Women between the onset of menstruation and the menopause should take three figs daily to maintain a proper balance of elements within the body.

Figs are supposed to aid quick recovery after prolonged illness. If taken in large quantities they can help thin people to put on weight. Body builders and wrestlers eat figs with nuts. Figs are also used as a laxative and are given to patients with constipation. And they help cure piles.

The skin of dry figs is very tough so it is better to clean them and soak them overnight before use. The water in which they are soaked also should be used because of its rich mineral and sugar content. The skin can be discarded in both fresh and dried soaked figs, the seeds and pulp should be thoroughly masticated.

GRAPES: The grape is one of the oldest and most delicious fruits known to mankind principally because it is so rich in glucose and because of its semi-acid nature. The acids and the glucose are thoroughly assimilated by the body and stimulate the activity of the bowels and kidneys.

The well-known Indian Ayurvedic scholar Vagbhatta considers grapes to be laxative and diuretic. The wise master Sushrut considers them to be srutitive and he believes that they provide the body with a life force which saves it from infection and deterioration. Grapes definitely help the intestines, and those who have weak intestines should eat a lot of them. The cellulose of grapes forms the initial pulp for stools. The skins should be thoroughly masticated otherwise it will produce flatulence. The acid of grapes cleans the intestines. Their glucose and sugar content is easily assimilated and therefore they are valuable for those who desire purification of the intestines. Grapes have also been found to be helpful in diseases of the skin and lungs, in gout, rheumatism, arthritis and obesity. Apart from glucose and acid the grape contains vitamins, phosphorous, calcium, some minerals, a negligible amount of fat and very little protein.

In India grapes are eaten both fresh and dried. Fresh grapes are either eaten raw or are used in certain exotic drinks. Dry grapes are of two kinds: (1) Raisins and (2) Munnaqua. Raisins are made from small grapes and are sweet and sour in taste. Munnaqua is made from large, ripe, sweet grapes and is sweet in taste. Munnaqua are very good for one and often they are recommended by medical people. They are very tasty and nutritious. Their glucose is predigested food and readily absorbed by the body. It enters into the blood stream as soon as it reaches the body and it gets converted into heat and energy within a very short period. Therefore Munnaqua is given to people suffering from fever, anaemia, general weakness, weak digestion, constipation, dropsy, dysentery, colitis, bronchitis, cardiac disorders and kidney trouble.

Fasting on grapes, or grapes and milk for four to six days once a year is a great purification. One should consume two to four pounds of grapes per day (±800 grams) during this period. Ripe, sweet grapes should be eaten fresh or taken as juice.

Vinegar made from grape juice of the sour variety is also good taken in small quantities with food for those who have weak intestines, weak digestive fire or who suffer from the humour wind, and rheumatism, gout and arthritis.

Grapes are an ideal food for children, young people, adults and old people whether healthy or sick.

GRAPEFRUITS: Grapefruit, a great appetizer and a refreshing fruit, belongs to the family of citrus fruits. Grapefruit was developed from a big, sweet lemontree which grows all over India. But the use of grapefruits in India is recent and they are grown only in Panjab and Uttar Pradesh.

Grapefruits are a good substitute for oranges and have almost the same food value. They contain minerals, calcium, phosphorus, iron, protein and a negligible amount of fat. They are an important source of vitamin C and E. Grapefruits balance the acid reactions of different foods and they relieve constipation, for that the fruit is eaten fresh with its pulp. Grapefruits ensure healthy intestines and prevent diarrhoea, dysentery, and other infectious diseases of the digestive tract. Grapefruit has also been found useful in various liver diseases.

Grapefruit should be used as an appetizer before food is taken and not after. It the juice is taken, the pulp should be taken with it. The varieties of grapefruit without seeds are healthier and should be chosen.

Fasting on grapefruit juice with pulp for three days is a great way to purify the stomach and intestines, because grapefruits in their postdigestive state produce an alkaline residue, although they are acidic fruits.

Grapefruit can also make fantastic chutney with mint leaves, ground with green or red peppers and with a pinch of salt and some freshly ground coconut powder. (Coconut powder is optional, one can mix it to increase the food value and bulk.)

Also a kind of salad can be made with onions, tomatoes, salad leaves and grapefruit.

Grapefruits make an ideal drink during summer. The drink can be made either with the pure juice alone or by mixing some raw sugar or honey to it.

LEMON: The lemon belongs to the family of citrus fruits and is highly praised in the Indian Ayurveda for its qualities. It is an appetizer and a stimulant of the digestive process and the process of assimilation. It is a healer, a calmer, and a nutrient. Almost every part of it is used for human consumption. Its juice is commonly used and the peels are used for making pickle. Lemon is of great medicinal value as a pickle (not usually the ones selling in the market however). In all stomach disorders lemon pickle is used as a home remedy. And lemon pickle is supposed to increase in medicinal value as it matures. Some sort of pickle is a must with food. Pickles tickle the tongue and encourage digestive juice and saliva. Lemon pickle is an ideal way of preserving lemon and of increasing its medicinal value. It is good to take pickle with the midday meal, but to avoid it at breakfast and dinner.

Lemons contain the vitamins C and P which has the advantage of making them anti-scorbutic and which prevents capillary fragility. Lemons also contain sodium, potassium, magnesium, calcium, iron, copper, phosphorous, sulphur, chlorine, riboflavin and nicotinic acid. They are an important source of citric acid and because of this they are popular in both medical and home remedies. Lemons relieve thirst, they are cooling, they relieve an irritable stomach, soothe the nerves and cure nausea. They are used for curing indigestion, acidity dysentery and diarrhoea of the kind where loose motions are passed repeatedly. Lemon juice is a sedative for the heart and reduces palpitations. The juice is helpful for blood pressure and for the bowels, the kidneys, the uterus and other parts of the body. Lemons stimulate the flow of saliva and cure the loss of appetite and dyspepsia.

Lemons encourage the secretion of bile and are therefore recommended to patients with jaundice. Because of its conversion into alkaline substances during its digestive action it cures all acid diseases like acidity, rheumatism and gout.

Lemon juice is an organic disinfectant causing no harm to the body tissues. It prevents the formation of stones in all parts of the body. Lemon juice stops colds because it possesses an anti-pneumonia substance. Lemon cures gas and its juice is a mild laxative. Lemon juice taken with lukewarm water every morning cures constipation. The use of lemon both in salads and as a preserver is well-known, but it is less known that people use its seeds. The seeds are especially useful in curing nausea when the patient vomits repeatedly and when vomiting does not stop in spite of several remedies. A few fresh lemon seeds pealed and ground to a fine paste in a mortar and pestle and then mixed with a teaspoon of honey act miraculously in numerous ways.

Lemon juice with a tablespoon of honey in lukewarm water taken early in the morning as the first drink of the day reduces fatness. Lemon is also used in fasting. To fast on lemon water for a week cures all diseases of the stomach and intestines.

In India a special lemon drink called *shikunji* is very popular during hot summer days. It is made by adding lemon juice from fresh lemons to a sugar solution. Some powdered spices with a pinch of black salt are then sprinkled over the drink.

Finely cut onions with lemon juice, a pinch of salt and a few freshly cut red or green peppers is a very popular salad amongst Muslims and onion-eating Hindus.

Using lemon with food, or in food, in drinks, as pickles or in any other way is good as its constant use keeps the body in good shape. In all preparations though always the seeds should be removed. The seeds are only to be used separately as the miraculous medicine for nausea.

The Spice for the Lemon drink shikunji

Take

(1) Two tablespoon of cumin powder, made from equal proportions of roasted and unroasted cumin seeds.

(2) ¼ tablespoon black pepper.

(3) Four to six cloves.

(4) Two red cardamom seeds and two green cardamom seeds.

(5) Two grams of black salt.

This powdery mixture can be made and stored in a glass jar which has an airtight lid. Sprinkle a pinch of it on the lemon drink, it has a good flavour and makes the drink more digestive.

MANGO: Mangoes are hot, unctuous, energetic and satisfying. A mango which has no fibre is heavy, though it tastes better than one with fibre. A mango which has more juice and also sweet, is very easily digested and provides energy to the stomach. A sour mango should never be eaten, except as the spice amchur (mango powder) and as dried mango flakes.

A mango which is ripe, sweet and juicy produces a lot of blood. If a glass of lukewarm milk is taken after a mango, it gives energy to the whole system and specially to the intestines. If, instead of a glass of milk, a cold drink made from milk by adding water to cool the milk, is taken during the hot season or summer, it reduces the effects of heat and gives strength, vigour and vitality to the system.

Mango excites and energizes the nervous system, increases weight, cures constipation, activates the kidneys and brings more urine through which the system is able to flush out toxins from inside the body.

Mango should never be eaten on an empty stomach. Mango keeps one young and helps one retain one's youth for a long time. Mangoes check premature ageing and hold back decay and old age. If one lives on mango and milk for two months — when mangoes are in season — one rejuvenates the stomach and intestines, and increases digestive heat and appetite. A drink made of mango juice and milk (the juice should be taken from a mango which has a lot of fibre and juice) is a cure for people who suffer from too little digestive heat, chronic dysentery and constipation.

Only juicy and fibrous mangoes are easy to digest. The sweet and pulpy varieties are hard to digest. Mangoes put into sugar-syrup and allowed to soak in it give energy; they are a tonic for the brain, stomach, lungs and blood, and remove constipation.

PAPAYA: Soft, sweet and ripe papaya is a delicacy. Papaya is considered to be a rich source of vitamins; especially of vitamin A. Papaya contains protein, calcium, phosphorous, iron and the vitamin C which increases as the fruit ripens and becomes sweeter. It also contains thiamin, riboflavin and a small amount of niacin. The carbohydrate of papaya contains mainly invert sugar which is readily absorbed into the blood. As the papaya fruit is exposed to the sun it gets sweeter and richer in vitamins.

Indian Ayurvedic doctors and Hakims prescribe the papaya to people suffering from liver trouble, heart trouble and intestinal trouble. The fruit is also used as a cure for worms in the intestine. The papaya encourages appetite, it helps digestion, it increases the flow of urine as it is a diuretic fruit and it prevents flatulence. The raw papaya is used as either a vegetable curry, a dry vegetable, or as delicious sweet dishes. Papaya has a good effect on the stomach and pancreas. It is used with meat and fish both, as a softener because it helps one digest meat and fish. Raw papaya converts milk into cheese and makes a delicious dish which is easy to digest and good for the intestines. Raw papaya is very helpful for patients with liver trouble, it also makes the muscle fibres of the womb contract thus aiding menstruational flow. But raw papaya can induce abortion if taken by pregnant women.

Ripe papayas eaten with cream, nuts and seeds are excellent for a summertime breakfast. In winter papayas should be eaten during the day and not after sunset. During the rainy season papayas should be eaten less because of their diuretic effect.

PEACHES: Peaches are cold and unctuous, satisfying and good for those who suffer from loss of appetite because of excessive heat in the system. Patients with fever feel energetic if one peach is given to them every two hours during the day. Peaches are specially good for bile dominated people. But because they also contain a sour taste, besides being sweet, they should be avoided by young males, spiritual aspirants and celibates. Yet eating two or three peaches a week is good for everybody. Peaches are delicious in a fruit salad with honey, nuts and seeds, or in muesli.

PINEAPPLE: Pineapple is cold and energizing. It cures anxiety and a disturbed heart and provides a cool feeling to the heart and head. Pineapple is sweet/sour in taste and sweet in action. The pulp of the pineapple quenches thirst and increases mucous. Pineapple is excellent for proper digestion when taken in small quantities with a meal.

PLUMS: The plum is cold and easily digestible. If eaten in small quantities plums produce blood, they open the lower digestive tract and clean the stomach. Plums are very useful in diseases caused by excited bile, or in diseases caused by excessive heat in the body. If plums are pickled in vinegar they are a fantastic appetizer and they help digesting food. Plums give strength to the liver and they purify the blood by expelling toxins from the body. They are eaten both dry and fresh. Dry plums are a medicine for fever. The sour plum is not good to eat, plums are sour only when they are unripe. If an unripe plum is kept for a few days it becomes ripe and then it can be eaten.

In vegetable dishes sour plums can be used instead of dried pomegranate seeds.

POMEGRANATE: Pomegranate is light, astringent and it subdues wind, bile and mucous. It is a palatable and unctuous fruit. Pomegranate is found in two varieties: the sweet one with small seeds and the sweet and sour one with big seeds. Both varieties are good for one's health. It is recommended though that only the sweet variety be used for eating purposes. The sweet and sour variety can be sundried and later used as a spice to give a sour taste to food and vegetables. The sweet variety of pomegranate is cooling and has a cold and wet effect. The sweet and sour variety is cold and dry.

Sweet pomegranates cure dysentery, diarrhoea, vomiting, dyspepsia and heartburn. They cleanse the mouth, throat, stomach and heart, increase semen, purify blood, remove restlessness and quench thirst. One pomegranate a day is more than sufficient. It should be swallowed whole and never chewed. In cases where heat has increased in the body both varieties of pomegranate will provide a cure. If taken in excess pomegranate creates constipation.

RAISINS: Raisins made from the best type of sweet, dry grapes are recommended. Not all grapes make good raisins. The high nutritive value of raisins has made them popular. Their sugar content is about eight times that of fresh grapes and their sugar is of as good a quality as that of grapes. The major part of their sugar is glucose and fruit sugar. This makes raisins the richest source of glucose. The positive effect of glucose is that it is readily assimilated into the blood, producing heat and energy which is the power behind physical existence. Glucose is used by the brain to activate the nervous system and it is the fuel for the motor which generates electromagnetic energy in the body. Glucose is therefore a life-substance that is regularly consumed by the body. Raisins and grapes are the best sources for glucose.

Since grapes are not available everywhere in every season, raisins therefore alone remain the main ever-available source of glucose. Anyone who is weak, old, or suffering from debility and diseases which slowly waste the body should eat raisins in some form or other. The iron content of raisins is easily assimilated into the body and they help the system produce more blood. Because raisins are more alkaline than many fruits they maintain the acid-based balance in the organism and provide one with more stamina and vitality.

Raisins are taken raw with roasted or unroasted almonds, cashews, pinyola's and pistachios. This makes a complete food which provides plenty of nourishment to growing boys and girls. This mixture is especially good for students. It is not advisable to use peanuts with this mixture, because peanuts are *tamasic* in nature, whereas the nuts and raisins are *sattvik*.

Raisins contain carbohydrate, protein, fat, calcium, phosphorous and iron and they also have thiamin and niacin. Raisins are an excellent natural laxative. The raisins which are made from the large variety of sweet grapes — the seedy kind — are constantly used by Ayurvedic medicine men and the on the Greek system oriented Hakims for medical purposes. These raisins are boiled with milk and given to a patient suffering from constipation, preferably just before he goes to sleep, so that the following morning he will be uncon-stipated. Raisins made of big, ripe and sweet grapes, called Munnaqua, act as a tonic for the heart. People can fast on Munnaqua alone for quite some time and even patients with chronic diseases can be cured by taking only munnaqua regularly for a particular period of time. Raisins facilitate the proper elimination of toxins from the body and improve the blood chemistry. Raisins make a fantastic combination with milk or yoghurt, because they both complement each other.

Raisins can be used in many ways, in curries, in salads, in breads, in milk, in yogurt, in sweet dishes, bakery and confectionery, in jams and jellies, in cakes, puddings, pies etc. The best way is to soak them for 24 hours, or at least overnight. Then the water can be drunk as it is or else added to food with raisins. The skins can be discarded if desired.

The water in which raisins have been mashed is a powerful tonic. It can be given to people of all ages. Soak the raisins before boiling them in water or milk. Wash them before soaking and clean them before washing.

In Ayurvedic and Greek systems the raisins known as Munnaqua are used more often than the smaller raisins.

Eating raisins daily makes one healthy and energetic.

Some Rules of Eating

1. Always wash face, hands and — if possible — feet before meals.
2. Never eat before sunrise or after sunset. If you must eat after sunset avoid all sour and acidic foods.
3. Meditate briefly just before eating (or offer grace) to raise energy and increase appreciation for food.
4. Always eat only when right nostril is operating; drink only when left is operating.
5. Eat or drink only when sitting down.
6. Never talk or laugh during meals — instead give full attention to tastes, textures and aromas of the food.
7. Always take water with a meal; beforehand if weight loss is desired, during meal if weight is to be maintained, and after meals if weight gain is desired.
8. Never drink items too hot or too cold. Water and other liquids should be served lukewarm.
9. Never mix temperatures in the same meal. Don't eat hot and cold items at the same sitting.

10. Eat only when hungry and after previous meals have been digested. Generally, don't eat within six hours of another meal.
11. Avoid all in-between meal snacks, including — if possible — all liquids but lukewarm water.
12. Never eat facing south — this drains energy and fosters anger. (East is best.)
13. Never eat unpalatable foods. This creates resistance in the system.
14. Eat only in a pleasing setting and from clean utensils.
15. Only take foods while hot and fresh. Reheated and canned foods create gas.
16. Eat neither too fast nor too slow. Don't rush and don't linger.
17. Avoid overly greasy and overly dry foods.
18. Whenever possible, laugh after meals. This helps digestion.
19. Never sleep within two hours after meals as this disturbs the mind and the digestive system.
20. Wash hands, face, mouth and eyes after meals.
21. Avoid all actions requiring physical or mental concentration for two to three hours after a full meal.
22. Urinate after eating — but do not defecate for three hours if possible. (Thus, one should not eat before his normal bowel movement.)
23. Never take hot milk before retiring.
24. Never take tea within a half-hour of meals, before or after.
25. Eat once or twice daily only — a light morning meal, if possible the main meal before sunset.

Sweeteners

Of all tastes, sweet and salty provide the common core around which most items of diet are created. In recent years great concern has arisen over sweeteners — which to use, how, how much, and how often?

Of all sweeteners, raw sugar serves the best in ordinary household cooking. Brown in colour — though not to be confused with brown sugar — what we call raw sugar comes from the second stage of the refining process. In addition to sucrose, raw sugar contains natural molasses in the unrefined state (as opposed to brown sugar, which is nothing more than refined white sugar to which refined molasses and other assorted compounds have been added). White sugar from any source is *tamasic*.

Honey is the pollen and juices of flowers which have been mixed with the saliva of the bee, which contains a wax easily digested by the human system. Of the various sweetening agents, only honey can be used in its purely natural form. However, this does *not* make honey suitable for cooking purposes, for when heated the wax is combusted and creates toxic residues harmful to the human system. *Honey should never be heated,* and thus should not be used in cooking or served in hot drinks.

Unfortunately for the unwary consumer, most of the honey available has already been heated, even those which claim to be "uncooked". A peculiarity in food packaging laws enable processors to heat honey high enough to combust the wax, and if this is done without bringing the mixture to a boil, the product can still be labelled "uncooked". Under these circumstances, the safest way to buy honey is directly from a beekeeper. If this is not possible, however, buy honey which has been packaged in clear glass containers and look for a sediment of wax. If the sediment is not visible, don't buy. Even if the container says "uncooked", the honey has been heated. However, if the container is labelled "unheated", the honey has been given no treatment and is safe.

Unheated honey contains a good quantity of this easily digested beeswax, which is pure caloric energy, heat in solid form which bursts into flame on ignition. Body heat dissolves the wax, but not to the point of oxidation. When consumed, this wax goes into the bloodstream and into the system — where it reaches the joints. Beeswax is the best lubricant for joints, and a powerful medicine in cases of arthritis and other disorders in which the joints are still or brittle. (A garbanzo-sized ball of beeswax taken each morning for 40 days greatly alleviates the suffering caused by chronically tense joints.) This wax also lubricates the digestive systems and tones up muscles.

Another marvellous property of pure unheated honey is that it can be taken with any medication without altering the qualities of the medicine in any form. In fact, the mixture of honey with many natural medications speeds their delivery to the affected part of the body, as well as providing directly usable energy.

SPECIAL NOTE: As a general rule, sweets should be avoided whenever possible. Sugars are the purest forms of caloric energy — throw sugar in a fire and see how readily it bursts into flame. This heat can damage the liver when taken in excess. (Alcohol is converted into sugars, and it is these sugars, not the alcohol itself, which are responsible for the liver ailments of the habitual drinker.)

Sugar is the food of the brain, and energizes whatever state of consciousness one is in at the moment the sugar is taken. If one is distraught, worried, anxious, or tense, sugar will amplify those effects. Confusion and sugar do not mix. Similarly, one should not offer any kind of sweet to a child who is on the verge of tears, for his state of anxiety will be increased with the addition of sugar to the brain.

In case of chronic tension, however, doses of sugar can be a valuable medicine. Two teaspoons of sugar dissolved in a glass of water with the juice of one lemon acts as a natural sedative. The solution should be taken only as necessary.

Both sugar and honey (except for medical preparations calling specifically for either one) can be readily eliminated from the diet. This step not only alleviates chronic anger, confusion and anxiety but also enables one to discover the natural taste of foods — and overcomes the dominance of the taste sense.

Antagonistic Foods

Certain foods, healthful when consumed alone, can combine with other foods to produce chemicals harmful to the body. Avoidance of these harmful combinations is a great aid to bodily health.

Of all foods, milk has the most antagonists. It should never be used in combination with any of the following:

Banana, green squash, lemon, oil, radish, salt, sesame candy and yogurt.

Yogurt should not be mixed with milk, banana, hot tea or any hot foods in general.

Honey mixed with any food above 160°F is harmful. Thus honey in tea, while tasty, is harmful. Honey is also bad with radish.

Buttermilk should never be mixed with banana.

Ten

Fasting : Reprogramming The Organism

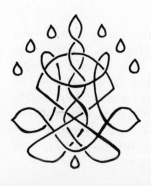

Food, sleep and sex — this triad may be considered the three pillars of life, comprising the common denominators which unite all men with each other and, indeed, with all life forms. From single-celled microbe to giant sequoia, all life forms take in nutriments from outside their systems; all require periods of rest during which metabolic activity drops enabling the regenerative process to take place without interruption; and all require a means of reproduction, of self-perpetuation.

No one can deny the necessity of this all-important triad. What can be questioned, however, is the amount and quality of each necessary for health and well-being.

The average man can survive 40 days without solid food, many days without sleep and a lifetime without sex. And there are those exceptional few who do not eat; others whose eyes never close in slumber; and many who abstain from sexual contact. How much food is essential for physical survival? How much sleep is needed for physical and mental rejuvenation? How much sex is really necessary? And, more significantly, how do these factors relate to each other, and to the physical and mental well-being of the individual?

There can be no absolute, general answer to these questions. The needs of each individual system vary according to genetic and environmental factors. Yet there are few in America who could not live as well or better with less food, fewer hours of sleep and less sexual contact.

How then can one determine his own needs? From childhood one is instilled with the "necessity of three square meals a day and a good eight hours of sleep." Similarly, the need for sexual contact, while clouded with the pall of "original sin", is acknowledged by all creeds but the Shakers.

The practice of fasting evolved as a means of self-understanding. For only by the act of volitional denial of a fundamental urge can its effects be clearly understood, and from this understanding one can then reprogram his behaviour more in accord with his real needs. Accordingly, there are specific practices for fasting from food, sleep and sex — and a fourth practice for dealing with the uniquely human ego: speech fasting.

Food Fasts

Food fasts can be divided into three categories, based on the motivation for undertaking the fast. Purification fasts are undertaken to cleanse the system, as a "tonic". Healing fasts are undertaken to rid the system of a specific disorder. Austerity fasts are undertaken solely for the purpose of denial of bodily urges, exemplified by the prolonged fasts practised by *yogis*. Because our main concern is self-synchronization, the focus here will be on healing and purification fasts.

. Take no food other than the single item selected for the fast.

2. Eat at regular intervals.

3. Never hurry over your meal as this disturbs body chemistry. Instead, before taking the food or drink, stop for a moment to recall the purpose of the discipline. Then take the meal calmly, devoting full attention to the act of eating.

4. No drugs of any sort should be taken into the system, including tobacco. The intake of drugs defeats the purpose of fasting, which is to restore chemical balance to the system.

5. Following the third day avoid exposure to sudden changes in temperature. The system is rendered extremely sensitive, and a cold or infection becomes difficult to handle after this point because no solid foods can be taken.

6. One should not lift any object weighing more than ten pounds after the third day. Normally, food in the digestive tract provides a cushion for the abdominal and thoracic muscles used in breathing, but after several days of fasting this cushion disappears, leaving the musculature to bear all wear and force without support. Lifting in this condition can cause severe muscular strain, even hernias.

This same emptiness of the digestive tract makes the respiratory muscles work harder, giving them new strength to work through old patterns. Fasting provides an excellent way of developing new, more effective breath patterns.

7. Feelings of weakness and dizziness are to be expected as the fast continues, brought on by the reduction of blood sugar. To compensate, one may take small quantities of raw sugar or honey — the total intake not to exceed two to three tablespoon daily.

8. Any strenuous physical activity, including sex contact, should be avoided. The systemic bal

Healing Fasts

To balance bodily energy and purify the digestive system *yogic* literature prescribes a specific program of fasting . . .

Throughout the year one consumes a bewildering variety of foodstuffs. Each food and each ingredient in each food must be understood as a chemical compound having particular effects on the system. Unless one is aware of and able to follow all the principles concerning right diet, regularity of meals, specific foods to avoid, manner of preparation, etc., body chemistry inevitably becomes imbalanced, opening the door to disease and suffering.

The easiest method of balancing the system is relaxation of the digestive tract by accommodating the organism to one single item of food intake for a prolonged period. Fasting of this type is best done at the time of the equinoxes and solstices for the sake of harmonizing with the ebb and flow of the seasons. The same food prepared in exactly the same manner and served exactly the same time for days on end provides stability of taste, texture, temperature, nutritional quality and chemical composition — enabling the body to accustom itself to a stable routine and begin the process of relaxation.

Naturally, the degree of relaxation is determined by the nature of the food taken. The basic food recommended, particularly when the system has been plagued by the various ailments associated with chronic gastritis and indigestion, is buttermilk prepared from yogurt according to the following recipe:

To two cups plain yogurt add an equal amount of crushed ice, mixing with a hand beater until all ice dissolves. Skim off and discard the white foam that forms (or mix with raw sugar and give as a treat to children). Now set the yogurt-ice water mixture aside.

In a metal ladle met one teaspoon of butter over a

medium flame. When the butter begins to sizzle add an eighth-teaspoon of cumin seeds and allow to brown completely. Now remove ladle from heat and add an eighth-teaspoon black pepper and a pinch each of asafoetida and black salt. (The latter two are available from Indian import stores. If not available, just add a pinch of table salt). While ladle is still hot, immerse completely in the yogurt-ice water mixture so that butter and spices rise to surface. Beat mixture again to thoroughly mix, then refrigerate.

This recipe makes about two quarts, more than enough for a day. The yogurt used should be homemade, and stored in the refrigerator for a day before using so that the culture has time to completely finish breaking down the milk nutrients. If possible, fresh, whole milk should be used to insure maximum benefit, but regular bottled milk will suffice.

No other food or liquid — including water — should be consumed for the duration of the fast, and the amount of buttermilk taken should not exceed a half-gallon in 24 hours. One may take as little as one or two eight-ounce glasses in a day. Additionally, the buttermilk should never be consumed after dark, or the danger of colds and infections will be greatly increased.

Yogurt is by nature a cold food. If heat is required by the system, one may take a mixture of one-half teaspoon honey and one-eighth teaspoon black pepper prepared according to the formula on page 195 (Black pepper section in Home Remedies).

This fast should not be attempted during the wintertime, in cold climates, or during the rainy season. Similarly, those individuals with respiratory ailments, as well as those extremely susceptible to colds and respiratory infections should under no circumstances attempt this fast. In these cases the freshly-made juice of beets or boiled beets may be used instead, prepared with the addition of the same spices.

The Virtues of Yogurt-Buttermilk

Hindu scriptures consider this buttermi Nectar of Life, a gift from the Gods to r good reason — buttermilk is a food wl anyone can take and which requires almc by the system to digest. All nutrients in t broken down by the yogurt culture, predige the chemicals needed by the system can p into the vital organs with little or no work of the body. The spices added to the mix strengthening the digestive system and settling acidity. Cumin additionally serves as a restor for kidneys and liver.

This preparation may be taken as part of tl diet, for it always serves to aid the functioni digestive tract. It is especially helpful for pa chronic kidney and liver ailments brought on indulgence in alcohol and sexual discharge.

During the Fast

The recommended term for a healing fast is fr 40 days. Seven days is the minimum period r for clearing the immediate effects of other food the system: three days to complete digestion, additional days to cleanse chemicals from bloodstream and the seventh day to enable the s to attain equilibrium.

The optimum time period is from 21 to 40 Fasting for this timespan not only cleanses the sy but allows the digestive tract ample time to recupe from damage inflicted by poor eating habits, overin gence in alcohol, excessive sexual discharge, irreg life schedule, and chronic disorders such as gastritis indigestion.

To ensure the greatest possible benefit from the f ne should observe several general principles:

becomes extremely delicate during prolonged fasting, and any exertion demanding a sudden expenditure of energy can wreck the harmony of the body and cause major disorders.

The Return Diet

The return from fasting is more crucial than the period of the fast itself. During this return period, one cardinal rule should be observed: take as long to come off the fast as the duration of the fast itself.

If one has fasted for seven days, the diet should be gradually expanded, returning to normal intake only after a full seven days. The purpose of fasting is to purify and heal the system. In the process of confining intake to one easily digested food, the intestinal tract is rejuvenated, replacing old, worn tissue with fresh, new growth. This newly formed tissue is extremely delicate and sensitive, much like that of a newborn, and should be treated accordingly.

After any fast in which no solid food has been taken, one should wait at least the equivalent of one-fourth the length of the fast period to prepare the system for solids. If one has fasted for seven days, no solids should be taken until the third day of the return; after 14-day fasts, one should wait at least four days, and so on.

On the first day of the return, one new liquid may be added to the diet. In the case of the yogurt-buttermilk fast, one may take the juice of one orange or lemon in a glass of lukewarm water with a pinch of black pepper, adding a teaspoon of honey if desired. This may be taken between the morning and evening glasses of buttermilk.

On the second day, another glass of juice and water may be added, eliminating the second buttermilk. The first glass of buttermilk should be taken daily until one has completely finished the recovery period — and in any case it is the best drink with which to start the day.

At the end of the first quarter, one may begin taking thin broths of boiled vegetables such as squash, tomatoes and stringbeans, seasoned lightly with salt, pepper and ginger. No solid particles should be left in the broth, which should be almost clear. During the remainder of this quarter, the amount and thickness of the broth may be gradually increased. Juice and buttermilk should remain part of the diet.

When taking the first meal with broth, one must take care to lie down on his left side for an hour immediately after finishing. This posture opens the right nostril, which greatly aids the digestive process. Broth constitutes a major change in diet, one which the system can handle only with effort. By remaining on the left side for a full hour the stomach has ample opportunity to digest the food without the diversion of energy elsewhere in the body.

One should not sleep during this time, otherwise gastric disturbances can result. In sleep the body's energies are concentrated in the head, and such a demand would hamper digestion and also cause gases to rise through the system to the brain, where they can create states of tension and anxiety. By remaining awake, energies remain concentrated in the stomach. For the duration of the return period one should observe at least 30 minutes of rest in this position after taking food.

Only after reaching the halfway point are solid foods gradually reintroduced into the diet. Only very thin soups of well-boiled, finely grated vegetables may be taken. Squash, turnips, tomatoes, potatoes and foods of similar textures should be used at first. Papaya boiled in milk and squash prepared in the same manner are excellent.

During the summer months another beneficial form of fasting may be practiced by subsisting on a diet consisting solely of one particular fresh fruit or vegetable, e.g., tomatoes, grapes, pomegranates, zucchini, pears, beans — generally any seasonably fresh crop. The main consideration is to confine food intake only to preparations made from that item of food, always prepared in the manner most readily assimilated and eliminated by the system. In cases where both juice and solid food can be prepared from the same staple, both may be taken.

The purpose of fasts of this nature is to attune the system to the temperature and atmospheric conditions then present in the immediate region. Throughout the year as different fruits and vegetables come into season for varying periods, any item may be selected, provided it is locally grown and available fresh and field-ripe. The item may be taken for the length of its period of ripeness.

One can continue this practice throughout the growing season, switching from one item to another as crops come and go. The consumption of locally grown food as it becomes ripe, attunes one to the vibrations of his own locality. In addition, this practice takes the greatest effort off the digestive system increasing the energy available for other jobs.

Fruits and vegetables ripen according to natural cycles and provide all the nutriments necessary for the human organism during the period of their ripeness. For this reason anyone would derive benefit from eating only fresh, locally grown foods. This is a general principle to follow in all cases of illness.

Cycles of Fasting

In order to harmonize the system with the seasons of the year, one should fast each year for a one-week period, during the same time period each year. If one attempts a long fast, in the range of 14 to 40 days, then the week-long fast should be done every year during the calendar period of the first week of the long fast. This habit establishes the system into the annual cycle.

There are also cycles of months and weeks, and it is these which form the harmony and beat of daily life. The week is a musical octave of seven notes, ending on the same note with which it began. Within the span of seven days one completes a full cycle of existence. Second only to the 24-hour cycle of the day, the week unites all men in a common pattern of life. And as one should fast at least once during the larger cycle of the solar year, so too should fasting be done one day of every seven.

All men recognise the need to give their muscles a rest from physical labor at least one day in seven; but fewer extend the same courtesy to their digestive tract. Yet the digestive system works as diligently in its own way as does the musculature of the limbs during hard physical labor. And if relaxation benefits the long muscles, the smooth muscles and glands of the inner system should derive a similar benefit.

For one day each week, therefore, one should abstain from all solid food, preferably taking only the yogurt-buttermilk or fruit juice. In this way the organs of the digestive tract can relax and recover from the effort expended in digesting meals the other six days of the week.

When should one fast? The best weekday for fasting is the day of the week on which one was born. Observing such a fast links one to the nature of energy which was present on the day of one's birth. Women, however, may choose to fast on Friday instead, a day when feminine energy is heightened. While fasting the system becomes more sensitive to energy patterns, and attuning to the energy of one's birth or of femininity for women brings one into closer harmony with his individual cycles.

Observing weekly fasts helps cure chronic disorders of the digestive system, lessens the desire to eat and promotes good health and longevity.

Speech Fasting

A man has just returned home from a pleasant evening stroll. Pleased with himself and with the day, he sits down to relax — letting his mind float freely. Within seconds he feels a sensation in the back of his head.

"Hmmm?" he muses to himself. "Now what can this be?" There is a thought forming, a feeling — something seeking the attention of his conscious mind. He relaxes again, and instantly comes a flash of recognition. "Aha, there is something I have to tell my wife . . . now what was it?"

"Of course — two people are coming for dinner tonight . . . That's what it is."

Now, thoroughly roused from his reverie, he calls out to his wife, "Cook something special tonight — we have company coming."

In this mundane example are recapitulated all the elements which govern human expression in each of its myriad forms. Encapsulated in this simple act of sharing knowledge is the very essence of the cosmic *Leela*.

Communication is a process of four distinct levels, ranging from the inexpressably subtle to the grossest expression.

All expression starts with a feeling, the sensation that something is seeking to force its way into the conscious mind. Something is there, but its nature remains a mystery. The evening stroller feels an insistent sensation in the back of his head . . . This is the state called *para* in Sanskrit — a word which means literally, "beyond". For expression at this point is beyond name and form. This is the stage of the "pregnant pause", when one is aware of something seeking birth as conscious thought, yet wholly unaware of its nature.

Then, almost immediately after the first sensation is experienced, comes the first moment of recognition, of identification. "Aha," the stroller exclaims to himself, "There's something I have to tell my wife . . ." The general nature of the thought form has been recognised. The process of definition and resolution has begin. At this level, where the first identification has been made — the generic nature determined — communication is called *pashyanti*.

Quickly now the specific character of the feeling emerges, taking form in words and thoughts specific to the experiences. "Of course — two people are coming for dinner . . ." Now the stroller has progressed from a vague and diffused feeling to a specific and discrete package of information, uniquely suited to one moment in space and time. Here, when experience of sensation has been further refined to the level of individual experience, communication has reached the stage which is called *madhyama*.

There is now but one stage left — framing and expressing the words in a form such that the one to whom the thought is expressed recognises it and responds in the desired manner. This fourth and final stage is called *vaikhri* . . . "Cook something special tonight — we have company coming . . ."

Now, if the act of communication is successful, the listener will recapitulate each of the four stages in reverse order.

The words are heard and recognised. People are coming for dinner. *Vaikhri*.

Then, muses the wife, I have to cook something. The words have taken on personal meaning. She has identified herself with the communication. *Madhyama*.

What should I cook, she wonders. She has to do something, but exactly what is still unclear. *Pashyanti*.

Now, leaving her mind open, she reflects. "Hmmm . . ." And she waits for an idea to emerge. *Para*.

The same principles operate in any form of human expression, from such everyday examples as that of the evening stroller to the finest creative acts of the most gifted artists. In all human creation the same play recurs, varying not at all in its general principles.

The composer feels something about to come. He knows not what it is. He opens up consciousness. The first inklings of its nature take shape. It is joy he feels, and that is the shape of what is to come.

Then the nature of the composition itself begins to unfold. It is a solo piece for an instrument, a vocal, a ballad . . .

Then the exact nature of the composition is unfolded as he expresses his feeling through the chosen idiom, the right medium. And if his work is successful, this same process is recapitulated in the mind of the listener. He hears the composition, recognises the nature of the musical form, feels the presence of a specific feeling — joy — and then releases himself into the state of feeling itself.

What is communicated in all instances is energy. For communication, expression, is the act of giving shape and form to energies which existed initially only at the most subtle and indefinable level of being. Communication progressively refines these energies from the level of abstract concept to concrete percept. And it is this same process which is at work in the creation of the Universe itself, as matter becomes progressively more and more defined from its primordial formless state.

In the process of individual evolution of energy which is *yoga*, one of the primary goals — indeed, *the* primary goal — is the elimination of gross frequencies of vibration so that consciousness is allowed to merge with progressively finer levels of vibration until finally all attachment to the base, material existence has been relinquished.

The reverse of this process is communication in which subtle energies are converted into gross. Thus one of the fundamental and most rigorous of *yogic* disciplines is the practice of *mauna,* of fasting from communication. In *mauna* all forms of communication are relinquished — not merely the spoken word as many have been lead to believe. Indeed, *mauna* is the most difficult of all disciplines for it involves quieting the mind completely, and allowing consciousness to merge into the state of pure *para*, beyond all thought forms.

Naturally, this is not a stage which can be easily attained, nor sustained for long periods. It lies beyond meditation, beyond concentration and beyond all action. To attain *para* the body must be in perfect tone, creating no disturbances. The mind must be perfectly stilled, with no thought-forming desires remaining. The attainment of *para* requires many years of training and strict self-discipline.

There are, however, intermediate stages, steps one can take before attaining full mastery of the mind/body unit. The most common of these is *mauna*, often called, "the silence".

Sound and Consciousness

The *mauna* is an effective means of concentrating, refining and elevating conscious energy. By maintaining silence for prolonged periods the nature of personality and of self-awareness undergoes major changes.

This is a technique especially indicated for extroverted personalities who seek to run from problems within their own character by imposing blame. It is therefore especially indicated for those who have undergone psychotherapy — which relies for the most part on the fixation of blame on parents or other environmental factors for individual character defects.

Mauna is valuable, however, for anyone who seeks to understand himself and the role communication plays in his life — especially the amount of needless energy wasted on conversation, and the myriad of other ways in which human expressions are communicated other than by word of mouth. It is a tool for understanding what has been aptly called "the silent language". And speech fasting is most significantly a magnificent tool for one who seeks to understand sound and its effect on human consciousness.

The importance of the spoken word in communication is self-evident. But few realize that the process of speech plays a crucial role in establishing and maintaining the body chemistry.

"It's not *what* you say — it's *how* you say it . . ." The most extreme threats may be voiced to an infant or animal, but if conveyed in soothing or unctuous tones, the response will usually be one of affection and acceptance. Emotional states transcend the limits of linguistic form. The purely sonic qualities of verbal communication convey the essential quality. Anger, joy, sorrow and contentment can be recognised from the sonic properties of speech alone — as anyone soon realises in the presence of those who speak a foreign tongue.

And coupled with the sounds are the arrangements of musculature used to produce them. The muscle set of an angry man who is producing sounds is readily identifiable, and the sounds share the tense and distorted qualities of the body musculature. An angry man looks and sounds angry regardless of the words he uses.

To produce different sounds, different sets of muscles are used. Each feeling excites sensation in different regions of the body. A man hungry for power feels "fire in his belly". One who is aroused by a sexual stimulus feels a stirring in his genital region. One who feels threatened "keeps a tight asshole", and one who is stirred to compassion finds his "heart is moved".

Similarly, the sounds produced in each of these states can be readily identified, regardless of the language used. A fiery speaker is a fiery speaker regardless of his idiom. A frightened man sounds the same in all tongues. The seducer's sibilant sighs are universal. And the sounds of a mother reunited after a long separation from an endangered child will touch the heart of any listener.

Sound and Psychic Energy

As mentioned above, different sets of muscles are used to produce different sounds. From the top of the head to the anus, the human body is a sound box, a resonator for verbal frequencies. This long column of air vibrates with each spoken word, though its energies are concentrated at the source of the sound's origin. For example, the word "lunge" expressed forcefully, produces a momentary constriction of the anal sphincter, and if the sound is prolonged, a perceptible tingling sensation will be experienced in the anus, which is the seat of the "la" sound. The sound "ma", however, originates in the heart — and explains why this literally heart-moving sound is the expression used for mother in most of the world's languages.

Extending this process through the range of the basic sounds produced by the human organism, it has been discovered that there are 52 key sounds which form the basic matrix from which all spoken sounds are formed. And each of these sound has a particular seat of origin, of vibration within the human organism.

Vibration is stimulation. When the flow of nerve energy to a limb is blocked, sensation is lost — the arm or leg has "gone to sleep". To restore function, one shakes — vibrates — the affected limb, and the flow of energy soon resumes its normal course. Sound production, by vibrating the body internally, creates similar changes in energy flow within the vital organs and glands.

As emotional states produce characteristic sounds, production of these same sounds can induce the emotional state with which they are associated. This fundamental principle has long been utilised by method actors and psychodramatists. By repeating "ha-ha-ha" over and over again, putting gradually more and more force into the sounds, one soon feels like engaging in genuine laughter. Similarly, prolonged groaning soon creates a feeling of genuine disturbance.

Emotional states are products of body chemistry. This fundamental truth is recognised both in Eastern *yoga* and Western psychopharmacology. Psychiatrists prescribe a chemical anti-depressant to patients who are brooding, knowing that by addition of a chemical to the system the feeling state will undergo changes. Mania — excessive exhilaration — is similarly treated by depressants. And so too for excessive sorrow, anger and other abnormally prolonged feeling states.

Each individual uses a particular range of sounds and sound frequencies. These sounds play a crucial role in maintaining personality by the recurrent vibration of specific glands and organs.

The human glandular system plays the primary role in setting and maintaining body chemistry, and it is these glands on which sound acts most directly and powerfully. Laughter stimulates the thymus. Humming stimulates the pineal. Groaning stimulates the anus. The sounds produced in most conversation stimulate the pineal and solar plexus.

The speech pattern of each individual is so unique that it creates electromagnetic patterns so easily discernible from person to person that they may be admitted as evidence in a court of law. This clearly indicates that muscular patterns hold true for prolonged periods, as well as the pattern of stimulation to the different ductless glands.

According to genetic factors (size of lungs, rib cage, voice box, etc.) and environmental factors (freedom of expression in infancy, amount of attention received, etc.) each person soon develops a particular set of sounds for fulfilling his personal desires. A "born salesman" is one who establishes a seductive sound pattern. The sounds of the "born leader" command response.

Producing specific sounds in the same manner recurrently maintains energy levels in the organism at the level of the glands and organs stimulated by those sounds. These glands and organs dictate body chemistry — and are accordingly responsible for both physical and mental well-being.

Personality can then be seen largely as a product of sound — especially when the personality becomes static, rigid and inflexible. And the process of altering or stopping altogether one's normal sound patterns creates changes within body chemistry — altering personality and ego.

Producing sounds designed to vibrate specific centres is the science of *Mantra*. Refraining from sounds to cease stimulation of habitually evoked centers is the science of *Madhyamika*.

Mantras can be learned only from a teacher skilled in their use, one who can best judge which sounds a student needs to produce — and only then guide him slowly and gradually into feeling the new patterns of nerves and muscles necessary to produce the sounds. No written text can convey this experiential information — and so our discussion of *mantra* ends at this point.

But, information relevant to *not* speaking can be expressed through the written word . . .

Speech Fasting : What to Do?

Who should speech fast? Anyone seriously interested in working with himself to create positive changes in his state of body chemistry. It is necessary to be able to refrain from sound production for the length of the fast, so a period should be chosen when no speech is necessary. There are only two conditions for beginning such a fast: desire and opportunity. Beyond that, there are levels of involvement, as with all self-disciplinary practices.

As with other forms of self-discipline, one should begin speech-fasting on a relatively low level in order to discover the kinds of situations likely to be confronted on more rigorous or prolonged endeavours. Initially, one may give up all spoken communication for a day. Gestures and notes may be used to express necessary information. The sound of slaughter may be retained.

The one-day fast provides an excellent demonstration of practicability. For some individuals prolonged speech fasts are impractical because of work or familial obliga-tions, and the one-day fast will soon allow one to discover if this is a discipline which may be followed. If the one-day fast proves successful, a few days should be allowed before attempting a longer fast. A three- to five-day experience may now be attempted, or even a full week. Again, allow some time for reflection and understanding following the fast. After one has become thoroughly acquainted with the nature and effects of speech fasting, there is no limit to the length this discipline may be practiced. There are religious orders East and West whose members voluntarily renounce speech for life.

But the abandonment of the spoken word is not the maximum extent of the possible austerities of this discipline. One can voluntarily abstain from all sounds, including laughter. Only the natural reflexes of cough-ing, sneezing, and belching are retained — and these should never be abandoned in any case.

One may also give up communication by the written word, confining expressions to gestures — and these too may be relinquished. But this latter course is virtually impossible for anyone who still has desires to fulfill in the world, and who must perform *karmas* in order to justify his existence.

The Effects

In prolonged silence, one soon discovers the extent to which most spoken communications are absolutely trivial, unessential for life, health or happiness. Most of the words uttered by men are "small talk", voiced solely for the purpose of affirmation of ego.

One also discovers that speech is a tremendous drain on energy. When one is silent and observing those who are not, it soon becomes apparent that excess speech creates excess *tamas* in the system. Talking tires, while silence rejuvenates.

The chemical effects caused by metabolic changes which follow the non-stimulation of verbally activated centers become apparent following the first ten to fourteen days. Sensory perception may undergo profound alterations as the system re-establishes itself in a new pattern. The effects produced are not dissimilar to certain forms of mild intoxication.

The desire for expression remains even after the normal form of expression has been abandoned. One soon begins to seek other outlets for self-expression. Speech fasting accordingly stimulates long-dormant areas of self — including creative writing, poetry and essays in the verbal realm. More significantly, non-verbal areas of expression are also opened up, including the fine arts and music. For one who wishes to learn music, drawing, painting or sculpting, *Mauna* provides a tremendous impetus in these directions.

By bringing consciousness from the verbal domain to the non-verbal realm, body chemistry is also altered. Verbal communication centers in the left hemisphere of the brain; non-verbal expression in the right. Each hemisphere operates through a different system of chemical reactions — as is explained in the chapter on breath.

Prolonged silence also enforces a continual re-evaluation of self. One can no longer express his identity to others through a show of words. His actions literally must speak for themselves. In turn, the reactions of others soon disclose in which areas his vibrations are right, and in which they are confused or disturbed.

The mind does not stop working merely because the lips cease articulating. All the thoughts continually flow by in the stream of consciousness. And because they cannot be verbally expressed in the immediate feedback situation of day-to-day conversation, one gains a deep insight into the importance and non-importance, validity and invalidity of long-cherished ideas and beliefs.

One also discovers that those things which need to be said *are* said, that what needs to be communicated is communicated by others — and there is something working which transcends individual ego . . . These are but a few of the observations made by those who have experienced the effects of prolonged *Mauna*. The responses and reactions vary from individual to individual.

Coming Back

As with all fasts, the return aspect of the speech fast is fully as important as the period of abstinence. With speech fasting, however, there is one crucial difference: one needs to eat, one needs to sleep — but one really doesn't need to speak. And so the problem is that one may not wish to return. But if one is to live and work in the world, one must return — in fairness to himself and others.

When one has decided to resume speaking, he should be aware that his organs of speech have not been used for a prolonged period, and that their chemistry and structure have therefore undergone alteration. Accordingly, one should only begin to speak gradually and refrain from any loud or harsh sounds. The honey-pepper tonic is helpful if soreness develops (see Medicines).

If the fast has been sufficiently prolonged, one will be well able to gauge the need for speech in his life, and of the role of non-verbal factors in the communicative process as well.

The main consideration during the return is to speak, which may require conscious effort if silence has been long, but not excessively; to avoid heavy bursts of speech followed by long periods of silence. Beyond this, nothing much need be said. *Mauna* provides a tool for raising energy by changing sound patterns, and by changing the self-perspective. One cannot emerge from a long silence with the same concept of self with which he began the discipline.

One now has a clearer idea of where he needs to work on himself, and the nature of the work to be done. And it is here that the real value of this discipline lies. For objectivity is the first step toward detachment.

Sleep Fasting

The flow of man's consciousness is governed by a natural rhythm cycle. The beats of this movement are called the waking state, the sleep state and the deep sleep state. There is a fourth state as well, but this last state is the elusive altered state of consciousness sought by the practitioners of hard self-disciplines such as *yoga* and not part of the normal daily pattern of awareness.

All man's life is regulated by the cycle of the three basic states. Within this field comes another rhythm, the cycle of dreams, which repeats itself in all three states. The waking state sees dreams manifest as fantasies and day dreams; while the two sleeping states see dreams in their purest form.

Fantasies and daydreams consume more human energy than any other endeavour. Man has wasted more time on "could chasing" than in any other activity. Daydreams and fantasies seize upon the awareness and drain off the purest and most subtle forms of creative energy, yielding nothing of value in daily life.

Fantasies and daydreams are an escape from the world of action into the realm of self-indulgence. Fantasies are not imagination, for imagination implies conscious control of the creative faculties for the evolution of a specific goal. Fantasies are undirected manifestations of unfilled desires which yield no practical means of fulfilling desires. Imagination is the directed manifestation of an unfulfilled desire, focussed in the most effective manner to bring about fulfilment of the desire.

The constant barrage of sensory stimuli presented by the electronic and print media creates a multidate of desires, in turn triggering human fantasies at an unprecedented rate. As machines free man from hard labor and long working hours, the empty void of time thus created is filled with fantasy for too frequently.

To break this rhythm of consciousness and restore mind and body to a zero point from where to tune the clock of life in synchrony with the rhythm of the planet is the job of the sleep fast.

Man is consciousness, with five work organs and five sense organs at his disposal. Consciousness gives man purpose; the work organs and sense organs, the ability to fulfill his purpose. The real task confronting man is realization of his own true nature (pure consciousness) without falling into the snares created by his own tools.

Man's body is a vehicle. One has not to make the mistake of identifying the driver with the vehicle. Consciousness is the driver, and it is consciousness which has the free will to leave the vehicle. The vehicle, however, cannot move without the driver.

This perspective should be well understood, for otherwise man feels enslaved by his own body. The purpose of the sleep fast is to give man a real understanding about body, to educate him about his own lack of control over his own organs of perception and action.

Sleep fasting is work against gravity, and against the natural rhythms of the body — which are primarily governed by gravity. Because man lives of Earth, his body is made to work in accordance with the laws of Earth. And gravity is the first of laws for earthly life.

In sleep, the body surrenders each and every cell to the inexorable pull of mass attraction. Each and every square inch of the body feels the pull. The blood is able to flow uniformly and without great effort throughout the whole system, recharging and replenishing the tissues.

In standing and sitting, conversely, the body is at a right angle with the plane of the planet's surface. Less body area is directly exposed to gravity, and the column that is the spine stands erect and opposed to the natural pull of energy. Man is the only organism to spend most of his life with his spine straight and at direct odds with the natural pull of energy.

The entire human body functions through the spinal chord, the directing center for which is the brain. When kept at a 90 degree alignment with the Earth, the brain and spinal chord form an independent circuit. To hold the body in this position requires more energy, for the heart must push the blood upward, against the natural pull of gravity. And to hold the body erect requires alertness, for the slightest lapse into the dreaming and sleeping states create imbalance, and anything balanced on but two legs easily falls.

Sleep fasting works against gravity, and against the habitual rhythms of the human system. Sleep fasting works against the desires which dominate and enslave the human consciousness.

Food, sex and sleep are the three pillars on which the human organism is built. By controlling diet, one can also regulate his sexual and sleeping cycles. By controlling his sexual drives, one can regulate his diet and sleep pattern. And by controlling his desire to sleep, one can regulate both his sexuality and his diet. One who gains control of any one of these drives controls all three; and one who masters all three becomes master of the world.

To understand sleep fasting it is necessary to return to the perspective offered by an understanding of the three cosmic forces, the three *gunas*. Food is the element of *rajas* in human life, that which provides man with the energy and activity to realize his goal. Sleep is the *tamas*, the inertia, the surrender to mass. Sex — procreation — the *sattwa* of human life, the prime directive of all animate forms. Sleep helps the body balance itself and restore energy to all its parts. Food provides the energy without which all actions would become impossible. Sex gives birth to life, and without it no play would be possible on the stage of the world.

In sleep the whole world vanishes as the sense organs turn in open themselves and withdraw from the phenomenal world. The body has totally surrendered to gravity. One has become pure *tamas*.

One who reads and understands the section on *sattva*, *rajas* and *tamas* and bears this awareness constantly in mind will perceive everything in his own system as part of a coherent and meaningful whole — where all internal events have their external counterparts, and where there is no sense of alienation and separation. One who lacks this understanding sees a world which remains basically unrelated and incoherent.

One can only understand the nature of the three *gunas* by understanding and mastering them within his own system. Sleep fasting brings victory over *tamas*, and winning over *tamas* can only be achieved by action — for it is *rajas* which converts *tamas* into *sattva*, ignorance into understanding.

The Physiology of Sleep Fasting

When a physician wants to measure the activity taking place within the human brain he attaches small electrical conductors to the skull of his subject, and through them monitors the ceaseless rhythms of electrical energy ebbing and flowing within the skull.

Experiments have disclosed that the intensity of electrical activity increases when subjects are deprived of sleep. Consequently, it has become a general practice of physicians to keep their patients awake on the night before administering a recording of brainwaves.

Thus, as the evidence of the electroencephalograph shows, sleep fasting charges the brain and makes normally subtle and undetectable currents of energy apparent.

This fact is common knowledge to medical men, and to ascetics of all religious traditions. Unfortunately, it is neither known nor understood by the majority of men.

Normally, the body surrenders to *tamas* at night and the normal cycle of activity ceases. No energy is required by the sense organs or work organs, and this surplus can be used to recharge the system. The brain too gains a measure of relaxation, as no energy is required for conscious action (though the midbrain and brainstorm still must regulate autonomic functions, and the cortex may be engaged in dreaming).

In sleep fasting, there is more combustion taking place in the brain cells. Considerable energy must be expending in fighting the natural inclination to lie down and allow the mantle of *tamas* to extinguish the light of awareness. One is fighting against the natural patterned responses of the muscles, which are habituated to sleeping at night. This whole process also demands that consciousness keep itself continually engaged in some activity, for otherwise *tamas* takes over with the slightest lapse of attention. Consequently, the brain of one involved in sleep fasting is a beehive of electrical activity, as new directives continually override automatic programs and as the mind strives to keep itself engaged.

The normal muscular and nervous responses dictate sleep. The will of the sleep-faster dictates awareness. To keep aware, he must keep engaged, and engagement means concentration of sense organs and work organs. Thus energy is operating at many levels in the sleep fast, and at a greater intensity than in normal circumstances. This demand for energy creates more heat in the brain, as the nerve cells burn up glucose and protein at rates much higher than normal. This intense heat, in turn, produces a drying of the brain tissues. And this drying is the cause of a cleansing process which is one of the primary advantages of the sleep fast.

Whenever there is abnormal heat in any part of the body, the moisture in that area is consumed. To compensate for this imbalance, the system rushes new moisture to that region, to preserve the balance of life. In sleep fasting, dryness is created in the head, bringing a rush of new fluids to the brain. The old fluids are consumed, and along with them old chemical wastes are flushed out of the system, followed by a rush of fresh chemicals and new energy. Sleep fasting is similar to filling up a tank after first completely cleansing it by fire.

If sleep fasting is extended beyond one night, the amount of resistance required to overcome the ever-increasing desire to sleep must be continually expanded. More and more energy is required simply for staying awake. This is why lapses of memory are common following the third day of a sleep fast, followed not long afterwards by imbalance, loss of coordination, visual distortions and outright hallucinations. If continued through the seventh day, one may completely lose track of his sense organs and work organs.

Fasts extended beyond the seventh day can generate such heat in the brain that new circuits of activity are created and sleep becomes impossible. For this reason prolonged sleep fasts are destructive in nature, especially so when not carried out in the presence of one who has mastered this hazardous science. This insomnia which follows prolonged sleep fasting is the same insomnia which appears in cases of schizophrenia, and may be accompanied by the same distortions of reality.

Development of Will

Sleep fasts provide an important tool for improving the chemical balance in the human brain. But of equal importance is the role fasting plays in developing the human faculties of will be determination.

By overcoming any of one's weaknesses, one gains the awareness and determination that other weaknesses can be overcome in their turn. The only thing which prevents man from overcoming his own failings in weakness and indecision. By mastering one weakness, the system creates within itself the understanding that every job can be handled in the same manner. This understanding is called *will*.

By exercise of the will time and time again, one gains strength of character — and strength of character and strength of will are in reality indistinguishable. The whole psychodrama of human existence is based on the interplay of will and desire. Desires are a network of sensory stimuli which trigger the faculty of memory and stimulate electrical activity in the brain. Will is the computer that analyzes the nature of the desires and, with the help of the memory bank of individual and racial experience filters out all factors and based on them returns a positive, negative or indeterminate (confused) signal to the body. This is why man, with the presentation of each new sensory stimulus, either moves towards the sense object, away from the sense object, or merely stands by in indecision and confusion.

Sleep fasting makes a man confront each of the elements in this interplay of desire and will many times in the course of the night, all in a clear and understandable fashion.

Man experiences the desire to sleep, his decision not to sleep, his desire not to sleep — and then the whole logical train which follows the question "to sleep or not to sleep?" Then, if his system permits, he feels the exercise of will which comes with the ability to overcome sleep.

A man desires to sleep, and then remembers he has decided not to sleep. Still, the pull of sleep makes him debate with himself for a moment. Finally, sensing that the debate itself is an enticement towards sleep, he does the only thing which can keep sleep away — he involves himself in an activity which is strong enough to keep consciousness engaged.

Man has exercised will — and more than that, he

had learned something about his own system of values. When sleep comes, all sense objects, all thoughts, all feelings, all relationships lose their meaning. To keep awake, one must find an activity to involve himself with, and only those activities which hold a high intrinsic value are sufficient to overcome the almost overwhelming pull of *tamas*.

The sleep fast is also an excellent device to monitor physical health, for the body must exert considerable effort to maintain itself erect and against the pull of gravity. In this process, fatigue may set in, and it is not uncommon to feel pain at different parts of the body. These areas of pain are the weak spots in the body, those areas which are in need of remedy. This is a particularly effective way of finding out about disturbances of the body's gases. Sleep fasting also reveals the nature of the cycles of the night, when energy goes through four specific stages as the planet rotates on its axis.

When to Sleep Fast

Sleep fasting can be done anytime a man desires, but as for virtually all human activities, there are times when this discipline will have the greatest effect. The two most effective times to keep awake are the Full Moon and Darkest Nights. These two nights are *the* sleep fast nights for one who is anxious to synchronize himself with the natural rhythm cycle of the planet. Other nights on which one decides to sleep fast are largely matters of individual choice and convenience, to satisfy any of the sense organs or the mind.

The Full Moon night has a profound effect on human behaviour, and on the behaviour of all water on the planet — as policemen, psychologists, security departments and navigators can all attest. The Darkest Night is the low tide time for both emotions and oceans. The role of water in the body has already been discussed in relation to the phases of the Moon in the chapter on the Science of Breath.

After the bright and dark nights, sunrise brings a new cycle of energy on the planet. With the descending moon cycle, starting on the sunrise following Full Moon, comes an increase in solar energy on the planet. Dark Night heralds the start of a cycle marked by an increase in lunar energy. During the solar-dominated cycle, energy is more concentrated in the left hemisphere of the brain and the right side of the body; during the lunar-dominated cycle, energy concentrates more in the right brain hemisphere and left half of the body.

To mark this change in energy by remaining fully conscious enables one to charge his system with the kind of energy which will predominate on the planet for the succeeding fortnight. It is for this reason that sleep fasts are especially prescribed on the Darkest and Full Moon nights.

Two other nights linked with the Moon cycle also afford an opportunity for sleep fasting in a way which harmonizes the organism with the cycles of nature. First is the eleventh night of the ascending Moon cycle, shortly before Full Moon. This night is especially praised by Indian saints and *yogis,* and the Indian system of medicine reports that medicinal and healing herbs grow most rapidly on this night. The second night is the ninth night of the descending cycle, approaching the Darkest Night. It is on this night that poisonous and toxic plants grow most rapidly and are at their greatest power. By sleep fasting on these night one synchronizes with the healing energies of the planets and avoids destructive influences during the course of the fortnight.

Sleep fasts can also be used for attaining higher states of consciousness, and as such constitute a form of *yoga.* Because food produces sleep, one who engages in a sleep fast has to eat less solids and subsist on a largely liquid diet. The liquid diet cleans the system, and the lack of bulk relaxes the digestive system and with it the whole body becomes more at ease. There is simultaneously reduced blood sugar, and more heat in the brain. This combination of stimuli leads to hallucinogenic states, visions and "mystical" experiences. In this state people receive "messages from God". This can be seen either as a true religious experience, or as an opening up of the system which has been purified by non-indulgence in food, sex and sleep. In this state of purity the nerves become opened up, and provide new insights and knowledge to consciousness.

Police forces have also employed sleep fasts as a means of breaking will power and extorting confessions. In extended sleep deprivation (which this practice is really is, for it is without the individual's consent), the same phenomena occur which occur in normal sleep fasting. Only in this circumstance they are exploited by the interrogators either for gaining the subject's knowledge of an event, or for making him believe something as true which did not, in fact, happen.

This type of sleep fasting breaks the will. When it is information the interrogators want, extended sleep deprivation actually makes a man either forget his resolve to keep silence, or to abandon it to the overwhelming urge to sleep. When it is "brainwashing" the captors are seeking — implanting false information — sleep deprivation renders the memory banks open to easy access and manipulation by skilled psychologists.

Because these phenomena can take palace during a sleep fast, it is therefore recommended that one undertaking an extended fast do so only in the company of those who share his own feelings and convictions. All brainwashing and manipulation is not intentional; and in the state of heightened receptivity which accompanies the sleep fast, the individual can create paranoid feelings in his own mind as the result of harmless words and gestures of others. This is less likely when the native is in the company of those he trusts and accepts.

Practice for Sleep Fasting

Following are some general principles for one who is attempting a sleep fast:

1. Avoid all meals after sunset. Eat lightly and keep away from any foods which are likely to produce gas.
2. Eat only once a day, so that the system expends the minimal possible effort in digestion — and so that less relaxation is needed to digest food.
3. Keep active, but avoiding activities which cause strain on the eyes.
4. Take rest — but only when wide awake and alert.
5. When feeling sleepy, move around. Get up, walk and move the body. This creates *rajas* and defeats *tamas*.
6. Use tea, if needed, in moderation. Stimulants are harmful to the system, especially when in a state of heightened sensitivity.
7. Never lie down. The only exception to this rule is following meals, when it is necessary to recline on one's left side for a few minutes.
8. Rest the eyes when feeling alert, but not when sleepy. Sleep fasting strains the eyes, and some rest is essential. Rosewater, mustard oil and honey may each be put in the eyes to cleanse them and protect vision (though mustard oil and honey both cause a temporary and sometimes painful stinging).
9. Avoid driving or riding in vehicles. Driving is dangerous, and even riding in a vehicle will produce sleep because of the vibrations the machinery and roadway produce.
10. Avoid all disquieting or discomforting individuals and influences.
11. Do not extend the fast when there is any strong pain in the body.
12. Following the fast, take only the usual amount of sleep on the first night. This insures that the effects

Similarly, the lymphatic system no longer has to fight the pull of gravity in its continual efforts to cleanse and nourish the system. And the nervous system, relieved of the countless commands dictated by a conscious system, also gains time to rest and recuperate.

Thus, in sleep the body is surcharged with inertia which it will consume in the following day's cycle of activity.

Circulation to the brain also increases, as the whole head is provided with more oxygen and vital force. It is for this reason that most people prefer to sleep with no coverings for their heads, even though the rest of the body be well covered.

Sleep, then, is a natural and essential process for rejuvenating the body, and in proper proportion can bring nothing but benefit. But sleep is only purely beneficial when not taken in excess, or too little. It is only through personal experimentation that one can find the sleep cycle which is right for himself.

There are, fortunately, a series of basic guidelines:

1. Persons who do hard manual labour need more sleep than those whose work requires less expenditure of physical stamina.
2. Persons involved in serving positions require more sleep than those in administrative positions.
3. Persons involved in administrative work need more sleep than those who have retired or withdrawn from worldly affairs.
4. Sleep needs also vary with age. A child in his first seven years requires 10 to 12 hours nightly. A child in his second seven years needs 8 to 10 hours. A youth in his third seven years requires 6 to 8 hours. A young man in his fourth seven years needs 5 to 6. One who has crossed his fourth seven years and entered his fifth requires 4 to 5 hours. A man in his sixth cycle must have 3 to 4 hours. A man in his seventh cycle requires very little sleep.

of the fast will remain with the system. Never, in any case, sleep beyond sunrise.

13. Do not attempt an extended fast if any social responsibilities must be met in that time. Behaviour and even appearance undergo changes during a sleep fast which can severely interfere with normal social functioning.

Who Should Not Sleep Fast

The following types of people should not attempt a sleep fast, even for one night: those suffering from gastritis or colitis; patients of indigestion; persons with weak or defective vision and other eye ailments (including color-blindness); children ten years of age and younger; those over 70 years of age. Sleep fasts are also harmful for anyone who has undertaken prolonged, exerting labour which demands physical rest. Similarly, one who has just completed a long journey should not sleep fast. In both these cases one needs an oil massage, lukewarm bath and a good night's sleep to restore proper energies.

Eleven

Notes On Sleep

Sleep is one of the least understood of human phenomena, a void broken by a few scarcely remembered dreams, which consumes up to a third of each lifespan.

Of the three pillars of human life — food, sex and sleep — only the effects of sleep are, by and large, purely beneficial. Oversleeping, while not desirable, is not nearly so harmful to the system as excessive loss of semen of frequent and too large meals.

Why do all animals, save the nocturnal carnivores, sleep at night? Clearly there is relationship between the cycle of the Sun and the cycle of sleep. During the course of any given day, half the planet is facing the Sun, half the planet faces interstellar blackness.

The gravitational pull on that half exposed to the Sun is less than that on the dark side, for the Sun's gravitational pull compensates in a very small way for the mass of the Earth when Sun is overhead. Similarly, when Sun is on the other side of the planet from where one is living, both Sun and Earth are pulling in the same direction — toward the mass of the planet.

The Sun is the giver of life, and during the continually bombards the planet with energizin tions — the frequencies which enable plants to waste gas to breathable air, which stage the who of weather and seasons, and which give man li work and play by. This same light is a powerful stim to pineal gland — the master gland which regulate whole endocrine system (which is, in turn, lar responsible for setting the pace of body chemistry). Li induces the pineal to produce serotonin, a stimula which triggers activity in the body.

By this combination of factors it becomes clear tha there is a major difference in the nature and intensity of energy present on the two halves of the planet, light and dark.

Solar energy is *rajas*, and where it is present creates activity on the planet. The dark half of the planet is dominated by *tamas*. In daylight men are active, the *rajas*-dominated state of consciousness, at night men sleep — the *tamas*-dominated state of consciousness.

When *tamas* dominates human consciousness, it brings on dullness, drowsiness, ignorance, lack of meaning and stupidity. One loses all inspiration, and the sense organs withdraw from the external realm to become perfectly introverted.

Sleep is a mechanism provided by nature to restore the inertia (*tamas*) of the body, the same *tamas* which is the food *rajas* used to create *sattva*. In sleep the spinal chord stretches out parallel to the plane of the Earth's surface, giving the maximum possible exposure of surface area to the direct pull of gravity.

The heart, which normally has to work to push blood upwards to head, neck, shoulders, arms and upper chest, can now pump blood throughout the system with a minimum effort. Thus, in sleep the heart — while never fully resting — gains a respite from the normal workload of the day.

It must be stressed that these figures are for *normal* human systems, not *average* ones — for normal is superhuman by average standards.

5. Regardless of age, one who has passed his 21st year should take no more than eight hours' sleep nightly. More sleep than this will create an excess of *tamas* in the system and cause one to feel tired and listless throughout the day.

There is one basic principle pertaining to sleep. If one feels refreshed and inspired after awakening, then the hours of sleep are properly regulated to the needs of his system. If one awakens feeling tired and drained, it is most likely that the period of sleep is too long. One should gradually reduce his sleeping time in 15-minute increments until he finds the cycle which awakens him with feelings of freshness and vitality.

Sleeping during the day disturbs gases, bile, lymph and blood flow. This practice creates disturbance of breathing, disorders of the chest region, heaviness in the head and many other disorders. Sleeping by day and working by night is an evil habit, too. However, those who are scheduled to work at night soon become accustomed to the practice, and for such persons (e.g., jazz musicians), it may be allowed.

Sleeping during the day is allowed for healthy persons who have done hard physical labour, for patients of pain, breath disorders and nausea. Day sleep (napping) is also permissible for patients of gastric disorders and alcoholic intoxication, and for those who are fasting from food and find sleep necessary. Naps are also good during the hottest part of the day in extremely warm climates, but only in a cool shady spot should rest be taken. *Yoga* texts, however, forbid all day sleep except in cases of illness.

The best hours for sleep are those from three hours after sunset to 90 minutes before dawn. Going to bed with a full stomach diverts energy from recharging the system and increases *tamas* in the system, as well as producing bad dreams.

In all cases, one should have fresh air in the room where he is sleeping. Taking rest in an unventilated room is very injurious to the system.

If one takes no sleep during the day, and never sleeps within three hours after eating, he will remain always young and charming, according to *Ayurvedic* texts. The following guidelines will also help towards attaining sound and healing sleep:

1. Sleep only on the left side.
2. Wash the feet before retiring, massaging with oil afterwards.
3. Practise breathing exercises and meditation for a few minutes before retiring.
4. Wear the fewest possible clothes during sleep, especially avoiding stockings.
5. Never sleep with the feet pointing towards the south.
6. Never sleep in the kitchen, nor keep eating materials in the sleeping room.
7. Don't cover the face during sleep. This habit of covering the face is very harmful, as it forces one to breathe his own deoxidized air.
8. Sleeping in the open during summer is very healthy, but if there is mist, fog, rain or excessive dampness one should not sleep without proper shelter.
9. The level of the bed from the ground should be at least 12 inches.
10. Sleeping on a damp or wet surface is very bad; sleeping on a comfortable surface is very good.
11. The level of the head should always be higher than that of the feet.
12. Sleeping on the back is injurious to the brain.
13. Sleeping when hungry is very injurious to health.
14. Sleeping under the Sun is very bad; sleeping under the Moon is very good.
15. Lack of sleep and sleep-fasting is very injurious to

health. It makes the system dry and weakens the fire of the stomach and thus impairs digestion. Sleep-fasting under proper guidance and in the right atmosphere builds up energy, but done alone and without good reason proves very harmful.

16. Regular sleeping habits increase health, wealth and vitality.

17. Early to bed, early to rise, makes a man healthy, wealthy and wise...

Sleeping at the time of sunset is especially harmful to the system, and as a regular practice is said to bring poverty. Eating at sunset also disturbs the system and impairs digestion. Lovemaking at this time is also bad, for defective children arise out of such conceptions. Reading at this time spoils the eyes and shortens life. Walking or driving at this time increases the likelihood of being in an accident.

Twelve

Your Need For Exercise

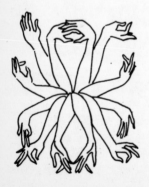

A life of harmony and tranquillity can be attained only if the physical organism is free from tension and at ease with itself. To achieve and then maintain the proper functioning of the body, exercise of some form must be practised. One is wise, however, to keep his objectives in mind when deciding upon the form of physical activity to be undertaken.

Exercise activities can be divided into two primary categories: physical culture and *yoga*. Physical culture has as its goal the development of a powerful, attractive and strongly muscled torso, and the mastery of the body by will power and nerve power.

Yoga, conversely, stresses *prana* — vital energy — and its proper flow throughout the system. The goal is not power and strength, but regularity and uniformity of energy distribution in the system, adequate for pursuing the needs and actions of daily life.

Physical culture trains and "educates" only the voluntary muscles of the body, developing them to their greatest physical capacity. Physical culture, moreover, is oriented towards the physical appearance of the body, the building of a pleasing external architecture. Thus, exhibitionism is inherent in all exercises of this type.

Yoga, however, has understood the human body far more incisively than any system of physical culture. It transcends the sphere of voluntary muscles by helping one gradually control the "involuntary" musculature — those bodily functions normally beyond conscious manipulation. And *yoga* additionally teaches that this control can be attained only after one has first mastered his breath.

Heartbeat is the key to the internal rhythms of the body, and it is the breath which is most directly linked to the heart rate. As breathing speed increases, so does the heart rate. As breath slows, the heart slows. Creating an even and harmonious balance in the heart and breath rates is the primary purpose of *yoga*. For when this pattern is established, endocrine gland secretion is altered and consciousness undergoes a major change.

The purpose of life is to be active, intelligent and inspired — endowed with fresh energy and the least possible amount of tension. Those who are physical culture fanatics invariably sleep longer, need more food, are generally dull and lazy, and accomplish less in life than those who follow the gentler, subtler discipline of *yoga*. Physical culture overworks the body and creates the need for rest. *Yoga* stimulates and invigorates, and its fundamental precept is: when tiredness begins, *yoga* should stop.

The highest purpose of physical exercise is the increase of energy in the bloodstream accompanied by a gentle increase in circulation in order to carry the heightened energy throughout all systems of the organism, refreshing and revitalizing the body. When performed in a systematic way, exercise harmonizes the breath rate, heart rate and circulation in a manner invigorating to body and inspiring to mind. The onset of tiredness indicates overtaxing of the heart and lungs. Exhaustion kills inspiration, while invigoration rids the body of wastes, the mind of confusion and the heart of burdens.

What Kind of Exercises?

Mild exercises are always beneficial. Strenuous exercises should only be performed for the express purpose of attaining extraordinary powers (*siddhis*) for the body. These and most other forms of *yoga* should only be learned from a knowledgeable teacher, one who can perceive the needs and limitations of the individual system. But while most *yogic* practices should not be attempted without instruction, one can always go for a walk, practise some basic stretching exercises and sit down to breathe properly.

The early morning walk is one of the most beneficial of all forms of exercise. Moving slowly and harmoniously with a deep, even pattern of breath synchronizes the whole body with the conditions of the day. A long, leisurely walk in the fresh morning air promotes mental clarity, physical relaxation, regular bowel movements and general well-being.

A general rule to follow at this time is: always keep the body well-covered from neck to thighs, being especially careful to protect it from sudden changes in temperature. The shock of transition from a warm room into cold air is the greatest source of colds, fevers and respiratory ailments. If the difference in temperature between indoors and outdoors is great, colds can be avoided by inserting cotton plugs into the ears and keeping the thorax well covered.

Walking too fast or with uneven paces disturbs body chemistry. Keeping the pace slow and the measure uniform allows the system to establish itself in a gentle rhythm which will last throughout the day. Running in the early morning, however, is the best hard exercise. At this time there is no movement, not a particle of dust stirs in the atmosphere, and the air is charged with vital energy. Running at a moderate speed with no haste in mind and no feeling of competition cleanses the whole nervous system and increases stamina, lung power and strength.

Deep breathing is the best form of exercise, one which anyone may practise. It should not be practised, however, before emptying the bowels. One should be seated comfortably with the spine erect. The stomach should be emptied of all air, so that with complete exhalation the muscles of the abdomen are drawn in, almost touching the spine. The sound of the breath should not be audible. Gasps, which are caused by sudden differences in pressure, can cause harm to the system and should never be produced.

The air should be drawn in through the left nostril, held, and exhaled through the right. The only time the air should be inhaled through the right is in cases of chronic chest constrictions. The flow can be regulated simply by using the right hand to alternately close the right and left nostrils. Inhale the air for one unit, hold in the lungs for four and exhale for two. The length of the unit varies according to individual capacity, but the proportion of one-four-two should remain the same. The air should be stopped in the nostrils, not in the lungs, allowing the ribs to be held open rather than locked. This is a practice which allows the muscles used in breathing to gradually break free of chronic "holding patterns", thus enabling the breath to come more deeply and evenly.

Other Forms of Exercise

When performing all forms of exercise, other than walking and deep breathing, two key principles should be kept in mind: the body should be allowed to move in the cycle in which it feels most comfortable and relaxed; and for each action performed, its opposite should also be performed to prevent any uneven development of the organism. Additionally, no exercise should be undertaken which disturbs the breath, causes increased feelings of tension, anxiety, pain or confusion, or which causes fatigue.

Generally, rhythmic movements are helpful for hands, feet and neck — slow twists, undulations, and circling motions. Sounds help the throat. Slow horizontal, vertical and circular movements stimulate the eyes. Deep breathing is beneficial for the whole system.

Those who are already established into some form of *yoga* should note that all exercises which bring an increase of blood to the head should be avoided during the daylight hours — this includes specifically the head stand and shoulder stand.

Who Should Exercise?

Exercise is beneficial to anyone under 40 years of age, for during these years the system is still establishing itself. When one has passed this age, however, only gentle forms of deep breathing and the morning walk should be practised. Exercising past the 40th birthday places a great strain on the system — as well as creating the foundation for senility and disease in old age.

Exercise is especially beneficial for those who eat a *sattvic* diet; most beneficial during Spring and Winter, helpful to those who lead a sedentary life; and of benefit to anyone whose breathing pattern is not deep and uniform.

One who desires true health should always reserve some time each day for exercise — but never beyond the point where the body begins to tire.

Who Should Not Exercise?

Those suffering from blood disorders, chronic cough or chest colds, and similar respiratory ailments should refrain from exercise. No one should exercise when feeling tired or confused. Similarly, no one should exercise within three hours of food, sex, heavy work or long travel. Those who are extremely thin and on low-fat or fat-free diets should also abstain. For these people only the morning walk is beneficial.

General Principles

1. One should never chew, bite or eat anything while exercising. After finishing with the exercises, if a real need for some nutriment is felt, one may take (after at least 30 minutes) some warm milk and nuts which have been roasted or soaked overnight in water and then ground well in a blender or on a rough stone.

2. Exercises should be stopped immediately when the mouth starts becoming dry, when one starts losing breath, or when sweat begins to come through the joints.

3. Males should always wear an athletic supporter during exercise to maintain testicles in the proper position, otherwise damage and infertility may result.

4. After completing the cycle of exercise, one should walk slowly at the same room temperature for several minutes, not engaging in any other activity for several minutes.

5. One should never leap into a bath following exercises; allow the system at least 30 minutes to re-establish itself in the normal cycle.

6. Following exercises, a light oil massage of hands and feet is always beneficial to aid circulation of blood and nervous energy to counteract the dryness produced by the physical labour.

7. One should always allow the natural instincts to guide his actions, considering conditions of time,

place, temperature, pressure, age, diet and health before any undertaking.

By following these few basic precepts one can establish for himself a daily pattern which will harmonize and regularize the system. One should begin any practice slowly, gradually expanding the scope only after the system has become conditioned and comfortable in the new patterns. By maintaining proper balance and proportion, a daily routine can be established which will greatly enhance both physical and psychic health.

Thirteen

Home Remedies

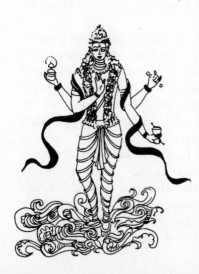

The system of medicine followed by the overwhelming majority of the Indian people has its roots in the principles of right living which have been handed down for generations.

Disease is not ascribed to the invasion of the body by micro-organisms from outside the system — but to an imbalance in body chemistry caused by a deficiency in diet, poor living habits or genetic (constitutional) predisposition. Bacteria and viruses may be present in the diseased body, but only because a disordered body chemistry has allowed them to flourish.

The organisms which modern medical science lists as the "cause" of most diseases can be found at any time in any human system — yet disease is present only in a few. How can this be if these organisms "cause" disease? Disease, and the presence of an unusual number of microbes, must then be considered as symptoms of a deeper imbalance.

What this ancient folk medicine seeks to do is to

treat both the immediate symptoms and the root causes which allowed the symptoms to develop. Accordingly, the greatest emphasis is placed on daily practices and right diet.

The adoption of two simple practices will keep the human system free of all diseases: rising every day well before the sun, and confining all food intake to one meal daily.

We have already discussed the great importance of rising before dawn. Confining one's diet to a single daily meal is equally important. This gives the digestive system ample time to thoroughly digest all food, and then rest. So often as a man eats, so often his energy is needed by the digestive tract to handle the process of breaking down food into usable components. Energy is drawn away from all other systems of the body, leaving one more prone to disease, dullness, drowsiness, fatigue, and depression.

One needs food to sustain life, but we frequently go without questioning the amount we eat. Supermarket shelves glitter with ornate displays of tempting snack foods. But man needs little to live on, far less than we are accustomed to believe.

It is an excellent practice to first eliminate snacks, then one meal, then another, until we are eating one or, at the most, two meals daily. This practice, combined with rising early in the morning, will provide a tremendous amount of energy and enable all jobs to be completed. Only those who are doing hard, physical labour need to eat more often.

These two basic practices, plus the additional procedures for daily living outlined in this volume should avert all diseases. However, the changes brought about by the adoption of these simple steps develop only through the course of time, slowly and gradually — so that until full balance is attained, some problems may develop along the way.

Because this is a handbook for daily life and not a medical text, we will confine this section to specific forms of treatment for relatively common ailments.

Types of Treatment

Indian texts divide medical treatments into three primary categories: *devi, manushi* and *asuri* — godly, human and diabolical.

Devi, the way of the Gods, relies on blessing, *mantra*-chanting, and "psychic" healing.

Manushi, the way of men, is the path of diet and medications.

Asuri, the demon's path, employs pain to cure pain. This category includes pricking, injecting, cutting (surgery) and shocking.

While surgical procedures and instruments are clearly described in the oldest texts, these are reserved as desperation measures. Fully 95% of surgical operations performed under the allopathic system would not be given consideration.

So of the three classes, *devi* and *manushi* are preferred. The most common forms of treatment include a combination of prayers, chants, *yantras* (visual centring devices), meditative practices, physical exercises (*Hatha Yoga* is part of this system), herbal medicines, dietary prescriptions and general living principles.

And because the prayers, chants and *yantras* are those of the Hindu tradition, we will confine ourselves here primarily to *manushi.* However, prayer and the chanting of songs from your own religious tradition can never cause harm — and may be a great help on the road to recovery.

To understand the way of *manushi,* consider the following paragraphs on the medicinal uses of the ordinary lemon.

Lemons: The Great Healer

Lemons rank among the most beneficial of foods known to man. Rich in citric acid and vitamin C, they are great aids to the digestive system. For gastric distress (gastritis), nausea, indigestion and diarrhoea, preparations based on this simple fruit offer remedy.

The medicinal use of lemons has long been a part of medical lore, as illustrated in the following folk-tale from Northern India:

Shortly before his graduation, a bright young medical student was approached by an elderly physician from a remote village. The healer informed the youth that he was getting on in years and needed an assistant to help him — and take over the busy practice upon his retirement.

The youth was delighted at the offer and immediately accepted, promising to leave as soon as his final credentials were issued.

On graduation day the new doctor gathered up his meagre belongings, loaded them onto a bullock-cart and started off on the journey to his new life.

As the aged buffalo slowly plodded down the dusty country road, the young medical man whiled away the hours building fantasies of the bright future ahead — an established practice, a comfortable income, and soon a wife, family, house, reputation and honour. A radiant new chapter was unfolding in his life.

But something he saw out of the corner of his eye jarred him out of his blissful reverie — a spot of bright green. Could it be? Yes, it was.

"Oh no," he moaned aloud. "I am surrounded by lemon groves. That must mean the village is a trading centre for lemons. And every idiot knows that where people eat lemons, sickness runs away."

His anxiety grew as each mile brought him closer

into ever-dense stands of lush green trees, heavily burdened with ripening yellow fruit.

His dreams of a few minutes before dissolved into a red haze of anger. His fists drew tight on the reins, his knuckles white.

By the time he reached the village his jaw was firmly clenched, and rage sent tremors running through his nerves. Indeed, such was his ire that when he reached the old physician's house he had forgotten all courtesy, all respect due the older man.

"What do you mean by this?" he demanded as he leapt from his cart.

The old man, sitting peacefully under a shade tree, stared in amazement. "Just what do *you* mean?" he retorted.

"Why did you call me here? What am I to do here? This infernal village stands surrounded by lemon trees, so what use has it for a doctor?"

He paused, seeing a look of perplexity on the old man's features.

"Don't you understand me? Don't you know that the Scriptures say that people who eat lemons never get sick? Why the *Shastras* say lemons are nature's perfect medicine and keep the system free of almost every disease."

A gleam of understanding shone from the old man's eye as he looked the angry man over. Smiling, he said, "Don't worry. There's nothing to be upset about."

"Nothing to be upset about?" asked the young man, for now it was his turn to be perplexed.

"Do you remember what the Scriptures say about eating the seeds of lemons?" asked the old doctor, smiling broadly now.

For a second the younger man stood immersed in thought, his anger gone.

"Yes," came the reply. "The *Shastras* say not to eat

them."*

The veteran practitioner chuckled, "I have lived here all my life, free from worry or want. And so you shall too. You see, people here eat the seeds."

Lemon Medicines:

Here are a few of the medicinal applications of the lemon, drawn from the treatises of *Ayurvedic* medicine:

1. For any acidity or gastritis: following morning centring activities, drink the juice of one lemon in a glass of lukewarm water. Add a pinch of black salt (available from Indian import stores) if possible.
2. For any stomach upset or indigestion: the juice of one lemon in a glass of warm water to which a quarter teaspoon of powdered, roasted cumin and a pinch each of black salt and freshly ground black pepper have been added. Use salt or honey to taste.
3. For nausea of all types: cut one lemon in half and heat both halves with open surface upon a hot frying pan until the juice inside the fruit boils. Sprinkle salt on one half, sugar on the other, and suck the juice from both.
4. For diarrhoea: heat the juice of one lemon to lukewarm, add the freshly squeezed juice of one lemon and a pinch of black pepper. Drink at once.
5. For severe gastritis conditions the following remedy is suggested:

    Fill a clay or glass crock with fresh, whole lemons which have first been washed in warm water and dried with a clean towel. Cover the lemons completely with crystalline (rock salt), cover tightly and

---

* Guava and pomegranate seeds (which should be swallowed whole), and tomato and pepper seeds are good for cleansing the system; but all bad tasting seeds are not. Lemon seeds are notoriously bitter and irritate the delicate tissues of the digestive system.

store in direct sunlight for 40 days, stirring daily with a perfectly dry, clean wooden spoon. After the 40 days, remove the lemons, wash and place in a clean crock. Now cover with honey (a natural preservative) and keep for use as needed. Take one-quarter lemon four times daily until condition improves.

6. One piece of lemon pickle daily, eaten with food, forestalls all stomach disorders. Here's the recipe:

Wash 25 lemons in warm water and clean with a dry cloth.

Now slice into one-eighth sections.

Juice half the sections, then place both juiced and unjuiced sections in a large clay or glass crock, keeping the juice aside.

Add the following spice mixture to the sections, stirring well:

One ounce ground cumin
One ounce ground coriander
One-half ounce black (red) cardamom, ground
One-quarter ounce freshly ground black pepper
One-eighth ounce nutmeg
Two tablespoons of salt
Four tablespoons sugar

Now add juice, stir and cover. Keep in direct sunlight for 40 days.

This medicine can only improve with age and stops the development of gastric troubles in the system. Be certain that no water or wet utensils are ever allowed to touch the mixture. If this happens, a mould is likely to form at the top. If mould develops, skim it off with a clean, dry spoon and discard all lemon pieces which have become discoloured — then replace in the sun until all traces disappear.

As a general rule lemons should be stored only in glass or ceramic containers. Never keep lemons on or in metal. Lemons, especially the juice, dissolve metallic oxides into solution — oxides which can be harmful to the system.

As with all foods, lemons are most beneficial when naturally ripened and grown without chemical additives, pesticides, colouring agents, and wax.

Here's another Indian folk-tale about lemons to illustrate the most common use of this excellent fruit:

There was once a young man who mastered the art of eating the finest of foods in the best of all inns and restaurants — all without paying a single shell.

What was his secret? The lemon, of course.

This young man would simply walk into a posh eating establishment and take his seat across from someone who was just about to be served.

Smiling, he would withdraw a lemon from a pouch at his waist. Then, with elaborate ritual, he would wash and dry the bright yellow fruit — all with an expression of intense concentration sure to arouse the interest of his mark. Finally, he would reach into his pouch again, draw out an ornately jewelled knife and with the precision and care of a master diamond cutter, slice the lemon in half — following of course a most careful scrutiny of the cutting plane.

By this time his mark would have received his plate. At this point we should mention that a meal in India is not complete without a good-sized helping of *dahl,* lentils. And *dahl,* like all beans, is notorious for producing gas.

His ritual through, the young man would offer half the lemon to his companion, a radiant smile on his face.

"Please", he would say in the most charming of voice, "have some lemon with your *dahl.* Lemon is nature's most wonderful food, and if you take the juice with your *dahl* you'll never be troubled with upset stomach or digestive problems. Please allow me to squeeze some onto your plate."

Flattered, the mark inevitably accepted, and equally inevitable was the conversation which followed.

"Aren't you eating now?"

"No, perhaps a little later."

"You must join me. You've been very gracious."

"Perhaps a little later — "

"I insist."

"Very well. If you insist, I would be most ungracious to do anything other than accept."

From this tale comes the colloquialism "lemon squeezer," the Indian equivalent of "sharp operator".

Black Pepper

Many renunciates live on a diet consisting wholly of seven black peppercorns a day, washed down with a glass of lukewarm water. How is this possible? Black pepper contains all the five elements in equal measure in a form which excites the body to recycle chemicals already present in the system so that no new foods are needed. For this reason *yogis* have long considered the lowly pepper one of nature's most perfect foods.

To prevent all diseases black peppers should be taken first thing after morning centring activities. They may be swallowed whole or ground and taken as a tonic mixed with honey.

To prepare the honey-pepper tonic, grind seven whole peppercorns to a fine powder and mix with a half-teaspoon of honey on a small saucer, mixing in a clockwise direction with the right ring finger. (Tantrics recommend 108 complete circuits while repeating the sound "Vishnu" silently to oneself, a practice said to further energize the tonic.)

Now take the mixture slowly, allowing it to dissolve in the mouth and filter down the throat — again saying "Vishnu" silently over and over until all of the mixture has been consumed. Avoid all hot food and drinks for at least five minutes to allow the system to absorb the preparation.

This mixture contains a thoroughly balanced form of *sattvic* energy and may be taken at the first sign of any disease — particularly colds and fevers. Mixing the two ingredients in the manner described literally atomizes the pepper, converting it to the form most readily assimilated by the digestive system.

This tonic may be taken daily, and is a great aid for promoting enhanced memory, greater vital energy, and good health.

Married persons may add a quarter teaspoon of clarified butter (ghee) before mixing. This combination increases sexual energy and stamina — and is therefore dangerous for those practising celibacy.

As with all spices, black pepper in excess can cause a disturbance in body chemistry. Too much pepper gives increased heat, anger, and dryness. No one should take more than the equivalent of nine peppercorns daily, except in cases of disease, at which time the honey-pepper tonic may be taken as frequently as four times daily.

Specific Treatments

Here are some Ayurvedic remedies for commonly encountered ailments and injuries...

Anemia, Weakness

Soak whole, fresh wheat kernels in a glass of water overnight. Strain the water into a glass and drink with a teaspoon of honey. This liquid is a great tonic and restores strength to the system. (This same water, mixed with a pinch of salt and a tablespoon of *ghee*, can be given to anyone who has ingested a poison, to induce vomiting. The chemicals contained in this remedy purify the digestive tract.)

The freshly prepared (*not* bottled) juices of beets and carrots increase blood production by the bone marrow and may be taken several times daily. These juices also stimulate the flow of electrical energy through the system and thus serve to combat the weakness associated with anemia. These two vegetables should be made staple dietary items of the anemic patient.

Anger

Expression of anger is a natural function — but only when merited by the situation. When anger becomes a chronic, habitual state, it creates a chemical imbalance in the system and must accordingly be regarded as a disease.

Hot (spicy) foods should be avoided by angry people, as should excessive amounts of sugar and heat-producing foods. Cooling foods, such as yogurt and squash, are best.

One-third of the juice of an average coconut taken as the first beverage of the morning for 40 days will cure chronic anger.

There are also several emergency measures which can be used as the situation merits:

1. Grind fresh clay, mix with water and roll into balls. Wrap the balls in a moist towel and keep for use as needed. Then, when anger develops, take two balls — one in each hand — and play with them. The clay absorbs all the energy and cools the system.

2. Place a few grains of uncooked white rice under the tongue and don't speak for ten minutes. The rice will immediately absorb all the anger.

3. Breathe in deeply through the nostrils and exhale through the mouth so as to produce a deep, humming sound.

4. Pucker the lips as though to whistle, but instead inhale deeply through the mouth so that the back of the throat feels cold. Continue this until anger vanishes.

In all cases of emotional disturbance, the breathing pattern will also be disturbed. At the first sign of anxiety and nervous tension, change the operating nostril and continue breathing through the new nostril until all traces of upset disappear.

Deep breathing is always helpful, especially during anxiety when the breath becomes shallow. To make this process more effective, always keep the mouth closed, fill the lungs completely and hum while exhaling — trying to produce deep, resonant tones like a bumblebee.

One may also produce a sound which is especially helpful for freeing the body of chemical produced in anxiety, anger and other similar psychic states. This is the sound "Ram". Fill the lungs completely with air, preferably inhaling through the right nostril. Then say "Rahhhhhhhh," exhaling all the deoxidized air from the lungs. When the air has been exhausted (and bad chemicals in vapour form along with it), close the lips and exhale the little air which always remains, while humming . . . "mmmmmmmmmmm."

Now inhale again through the nostrils and repeat the process for as long as necessary. "Rahhhhh . . . mmmmmmmmmmm." The "r" sound should be that of the Spanish "r" as in sombrero. The rolled "r" sound originates from the nerve plexus in the navel, the seat of feelings of anxiety and tension, and frees the nerves.

Other remedies for anxiety include:

1. Bathing in water which is below room temperature is also helpful, while swimming is especially beneficial.

2. Drink a glass of room temperature water to which the juice of a fresh lemon has been added.

Arthritis

Two medications have proven especially helpful for patients of arthritis:

One-half medium garlic clove swallowed whole with warm water an hour before morning food provides heat and lubrication to the joints. This should be practised daily for at least 40 days.

Buy pure, fresh beeswax and roll into 40 balls about the size of garbanzo beans (chickpeas). If possible, cover the balls with silver paper (an Indian medicine available from Bazaar of India), using one-half sheet per ball. Take one each morning with warm milk for 40 days.

Back Pains: Lumbago

To prevent and treat this disorder the following procedures should be implemented:

1. Eat regular meals, no more than twice daily, and avoid all in-between-meal snacks. Milk and fruits should only be taken with meals; tea or coffee a half-hour afterwards.
2. Avoid all cold and gas-producing foods. The following are prohibited: curds, yogurt, plantain, hydrogenated oils, peanut oil, fried foods, heavy dishes, chilled foods and iced drinks, canned food, stale food and reheated food, lentils, beans, rice, eggplant, cauliflower, etc.
3. Good foods to eat include fresh cow's milk, squash, rock salt, ginger, turmeric, bitter melon, cereals and light foods.
4. Eat only enough to satisfy half of the appetite.
5. Eat only at regular, established intervals.
6. Rest after meals, avoiding strenuous activities for at least two hours.
7. Never sleep during the day or within three hours of eating.
8. Use fomentations and massage (with salt in oil) as necessary. Warm water baths are also helpful — though warm water should never be used from neck up.

Bedsores, Skin Ulcerations

For bedsores and similar open skin infections, soak a cotton ball in mustard oil, remove, sprinkle with a few grains of salt and a few drops of water. Heat on a frying pan until the water sizzles, remove and allow to cool to tolerable temperature, then apply to sore. Mustard oil allows the maximum possible heat to penetrate the sore without producing cracking and dryness. Very little salt should be used — otherwise it creates intolerable pain and the patient cannot keep this fomentation on the sore.

The following ointment is also very good:

Heat one ounce of pure beeswax to melting. When the wax has melted add in this order: four ounces of mustard oil, two ounces of sesame oil, and two ounces of coconut oil. Do not heat to the point that the oils start sizzle.

After five minutes of cooking, remove from heat and allow to cool for three minutes. Now add one-quarter ounce of sandalwood oil (be certain to buy pure oil, not an essence) and pour into a wide-mouthed gas container. This ointment works miracles with bedsores and similar open infections.

Chest Constriction, Inhibited Breathing

For tightness and muscular ache in the chest region caused by disturbance of the gases, sprinkle freshly ground red cardamom seeds on two teaspoons of the skim of milk which has been allowed to simmer for an hour or more. Tension will vanish within five minutes.

For shortness of breath and other respiratory problems, stand by a body of water at sunrise to absorb ultraviolet radiation, a great help in these problems.

Other remedies include:

1. Fresh ginger juice and honey, one-half teaspoon each, taken up to three times daily as needed.
2. Boil eucalyptus leaves in a large pot. Once the steam begins to rise, cover the pot with a towel — leaving one opening from which the vapours can escape. Inhale these fumes deeply until

symptoms are relieved.

3. Massage the chest with a mixture of eucalyptus and mustard oils. Use two to five drops of eucalyptus oil to a half cup of mustard oil.
4. Bathe with warm water each morning, avoiding warm water on the head.
5. Hum during the early morning hours, creating bass sounds and sounds like a bumblebee.
6. Swim frequently to exercise and open the chest muscles.
7. Devote an hour each morning to sitting before a wood fire.
8. *Pranayama:* Inhale for one measure, hold the air in the lungs for four measures and exhale for two measures, gradually increasing the length of the measure. Inhale first with the right nostril, exhaling through the left.
9. The best treatment is said to be vomiting. Following the morning bowel movement, drink a pint or more lukewarm salt water and induce vomiting until stomach is empty. This opens the muscles and nerves of the chest region and is a great practice for treating cases of chronic asthma as well.
10. Never drink cold liquids — only lukewarm to hot; and avoid radishes.

Bad Odour of Mouth

1. Gurgle with water in which peels of pomegranate have been boiled.
2. Take 50 grams of rose water and squeeze half a lemon in it. Rinse the mouth with this mixture. It cures wounds of the gums, strengthens the gums — and removes bad odour of the mouth. (see also "Gum Inflammation")

Cataract

In the first stage, when cataract starts developing, use juice of lemon with a pinch of salt as an eye drop — twice a day for several days.

Chooran — Digestive System

Chooran is a powder used generally to improve the digestive system.

20 grams aniseeds — 20 grams oregano seeds — 1 gram of rock salt. Grind these to make a powder — add lemonjuice to make it a paste. Dry the paste and grind. Keep it in a bottle. Use one tea spoon of this dry powder with a glass of luke warm water.

Colitis (mucus in intestines)

Use thrice a day half a glass of fresh water with juice of half a lemon.

Cough and Asthma

To 10 grams of fresh ginger juice add 10 grams of honey — heat in hot water. Use the mixture twice a day for about 8 days. Avoid sour foods — including fruits and yogurt — in any form.

Cough

Take the skin of pomegranate — make a paste in mortar and pestle — add 20 grams of rock salt to the paste — and make small round balls of the size of a sweet pea. Dry them — and after they become dry — suck two of these tablets. Avoid use of sour foods including fruits.

Gum Inflammation

2 ½ grams of dry ginger powder should be taken with a glass of water once a day for four days.

Headache (caused by heat)

Peel zucchini and make a paste from the pulp. Apply it on the forehead of the patient.

Headache (old)

Cut one sweet apple — sprinkle a little rock salt — and eat it as first thing in the morning — chew it well. Avoid tea and coffee in the morning. Regular use for 15 days cures old headache.

Heart Burns

Squeeze one lemon in one glass of fresh water — and drink.

Improval of Memory

10 almonds soaked overnight should be peeled and ground into a fine paste in a mortar. Add to this paste 10 grams of unsalted butter — and 2 grams of rock sugar candy. Use it regularly for 30 days at least. This is a tonic for the brain, and improves memory. (see also "to improve Eyesight")

Inflammation of Throat

250 grams of juice squeezed from fresh white radish — and 10 grams of rock salt. This mixture should be heated together and used for gurgling.

Intestine troubles

Eat 2 ripe bananas with 250 grams of yogurt for a week. Avoid fried or spiced food and fat.

Jaundice

1. Take seeds from fresh sweet pomegranate. Keep them in an iron pot overnight in open air (better on the roof if it does not rain). In the morning add a little rock sugar candy powder — dissolve — and drink. Use of this remedy for 15-20 days cures all disorders causing jaundice.
2. Take fresh radishes with leaves. Take out the juice from the radish — and leaves — together. 125 grams of juice with 100 grams of raw sugar is one dose — and it should be taken once a day, only in the morning, regularly for 15-20 days. Avoid sugar foods including fruits.

Kidney pain

1. Add 10 grams of leaves from a grape vine to 50 grams of water — make a paste — sprinkle rock salt — strain — and give it to the patient. It relieves kidney pain immediately.
2. Heat the pulp of Zucchini after making a paste. Apply this bearably hot pulp on the afflicted area.

Kidney Stone

Take 20 grams of radish seeds and 20 grams of carrot seeds. Take a white radish, hollow it from the inside — put the seeds inside the hollow radish — close the hole with the same part which has been cut — put it in aluminium foil — and bake it in the oven. After the radish gets baked in the oven — let it cook — and take out the mixture of radish and carrot seeds from the inside of the hollow radish. Take 5 grams of these seeds twice a day (morning and evening). It is a strong diuretic — and will get the stone out in the urine.

Long hairs for ladies

Use one white radish with salt and black pepper every noon for 6 months regularly. It will improve the skin texture and make the hairs long.

Loss of Appetite

Five grams of ginger should be pounded, and a pinch of salt should be sprinkled on it. Use it one hour before eating for 8 days. Add some lemon juice if necessary. It will relieve the intestines of gases, improve appetite — and digestive system.

Males (vitality and vigour)

Take one ripe apple of the finest variety. Peel it, and prick in it as many cloves as possible. Keep this apple with cloves sticking inside it in a porcelain pot for a week. After 8 days take the cloves out, and throw the apple. Keep these cloves in a glass jar. Eat 4 cloves first thing in the morning with a glass of milk for 30 days.

Persons suffering from wet dreams or suffering from seminal diseases should not eat these cloves.

Avoid sexual intercourse for 30 days and do not eat sour foods — including fruits — for 30 days. Use the oil of cloves as prescribed below with the cloves for double benefit and curing disorders of penis.

10 grams of cloves should be burnt in 30 grams of chameli oil. The oil should be strained and kept in a bottle. Rub the oil on penis about 3 minutes every night, then tie a beetle leaf on the organ and sleep.

30 days massaging of the penis with this oil will make

the organ strong — and improve erection. Nerves which have become loose, will become right.

Menstruation

Boil well crushed carrot seeds in 250 grams of water until half of the water remains. Drink it adding some sugar. This mixture should be used regularly for two or three days. It helps the flow of the menses, and cleans the body.

Pain in Chest

Bake a few carrots in the oven — mash after they are cooked — put this in a piece of fresh clean cloth — squeeze — take out about 20 grams of juice from oven-baked carrots — add 10 grams of honey while juice is still warm — and lick it slowly.

Pain in Ears

Bake an onion in the oven. Squeeze — and take out the juice from the over-baked onion. Use it as ear drops.

Pain of Heart (Angina)

Mix a paste of 2 ripe bananas in 10 grams of honey.

Piles (bleeding)

Dry the peel of a sweet pomegranate and make a fine powder — use 5 grams of this power twice a day (once in the morning and once in the evening). Use this powder regularly for 10 days. Avoid hot and dry food.

Pus of Ears

Squeeze juice from sour grapes. When you have about 250 grams of juice — put this on a low flame in a porcelain pot — heat it till it becomes thick, like thin honey — store it in a bottle.

Whenever the trouble of pus in ears comes, mix this thick solution of sour grapes in a double amount of honey. Heat the mixture and put a few drops in the ear — every day for about a week. See if the trouble is completely gone. If not, continue till the pus is gone.

Skin of the Face

Beauty lotion: Filter twice the juice from fresh lemon about 20 grams in weight. Mix it with 20 grams of rose water and 20 grams of glycerine. Keep the mixture in a small bottle. Use it before sleeping on the face. Rub well and sleep. This lotion should be used for 20 days regularly. The skin of the face will become soft and beautiful. All pimples and black marks will disappear.

For removing roughness and for beauty: Take 20 grams carrot juice, 20 grams tomato juice, 20 grams orange juice, and 20 grams beet juice. Mix all above mentioned juices (they should be fresh). Two months of regular use of these juices cleans pimples, marks on the face, removes dryness, and makes the face bright, shining and beautiful.

Pimples: Take 10 grams of *malai* (cream) — squeeze 1/4 of a lemon — rub this on the face for about one month. It cures pimples and black marks on the face, makes the skin of the face soft, and provides it a shining lustre.

Spleen Disorder

Use the juice of one lemon with a pinch of rock salt for about a fortnight regularly. Avoid fried food.

Stomach Ache

1. Take 30 grams of pomegranate seeds — sprinkle salt — and add a pinch of black pepper. Chew them well and swallow.
2. Take oregano seeds 2 grams — cumin seeds 2 grams — rock salt 2 grams. Make a fine powder and squeeze half a lemon on it. Take the mixture and swallow it with a glass of luke warm water.

Strengthening Heart

1. Use 50 grams of apple jam (*Murrabba*) with silver leaves — every morning for 30 days.
2. Take 20 grams of raisins and a pinch of saffron. Soak the raisins and saffron in a clay pot with about a glass of water. Cover it with a thin cloth and leave it in the open air overnight.

   Eat the raisins in the morning as first food, and drink the water.

To Improve Eyesight

125 grams of almonds should be powdered dry with 125 grams of rock sugar candy and 125 grams of aniseeds, and divided into 40 doses. Each dose should be taken at night with a glass of warm milk. This will not only improve eyesight it will also provide strength to the brain, and will also improve memory.

To Reduce Fat

Drink the juice from one lemon in a glass of water every morning as first thing in the morning. At noon make a drink with 10 grams of honey in a half glass of water. Use this treatment 2 months in the summer.

Tonic for Speech Disorders

Almonds 60 grams — Cinnamon]
10 grams — Pistachios 25 grams
grams — Saffron 3 grams.

Grind the above mixture and mix with 100 grams
of honey. Divide it into 30 doses. Take once a day with
a glass of warm milk.

Tooth Ache

1. Take 2 grams of cloves and grind them into a
   powder — squeeze ¼ lemon on the powder. Rub
   this on the aching tooth.
2. Take 50 grams of the pulp of Zucchini — and 10
   grams of paste made out of garlic cloves. Add 2
   glasses of water and boil — until half of the water
   has evaporated. Remove it from the flame and
   strain it. Use it warm to rinse the mouth. Repeat
   this and finish the strained water from the above
   mentioned mixture. Use one mouth full each time
   and rinse it near the afflicted tooth.

Vomiting

1. Take one gram of cumin seeds and 1 gram of
   green cardamom seeds — grind them into a powder
   — add about 50 grams of water and squeeze half
   a lemon. Give it to the patient after every 2 hours.
2. Squeeze juice from a raw apple — add a pinch
   of rock salt — and drink.
3. 2 teaspoons of juice from fresh ginger should be
   added to 2 teaspoons of onion juice made from
   fresh onions. Mix well — and give to the patient.
   Stops vomiting.

Dreams

Dry the peel of a sweet pomegranate — make a fine powder — use 2 ½ grams of this power with water twice a day (morning and evening). Use it for 10 days regularly. Avoid sour foods — including fruits. Do not drink milk at night.

Whooping Cough

Boil the peel of pomegranate in ¼ kilo of milk. Drink it. It will cure whooping cough.

Worms in the Stomach

1. Drinking fresh carrot juice on an empty stomach every morning for 2 weeks regularly frees the stomach of worms.
2. Eat 2 sweet apples (peeled or unpeeled) every night for a week.
3. Use 2 tomatoes with salt and black pepper first thing every morning for a period of about 12-15 days.

Chronic Indigestion

Eating once or twice daily, never after sunset, and avoiding all in-between-meal snacks should relieve most chronic indigestion. Eat only when the right nostril is operating and lay on the left side for at least 20 minutes after meals. For those who can sit in the lotus posture, 30 minutes daily in this position while contemplating the navel will permanently resolve this problem in a few months. Fasting on either lemon juice and water or the yogurt-buttermilk is recommended — at least one day each week, preferably on the weekday of birth. Other remedies include:

1. One teaspoon of fresh grape wine 30 minutes

before meals.
2. A small amount of fresh pineapple after meals.
3. Vomiting once a month. Take a pint of lukewarm salt water after morning defecation and induce vomiting until the stomach is empty.
4. One-third the milk of an average coconut in the morning before breakfast as a regular practice.
5. A mixture of one-half teaspoon each of baking soda and oregano seeds (*ajwain*) with a dash of salt, chased with a glass of lukewarm water to alleviate immediate symptoms.
6. Reduce or eliminate the consumption of coffee, cigarettes and tea.
7. Drink the juice of one whole lemon each morning in a glass of lukewarm water.
8. Avoid rice, beans, lentils, cauliflower and eggplant — while increasing the use of buttermilk.
9. Avoid fried food, oils and butter.
10. Eat only half the usual meal, and only eat when very hungry.
11. Take breads made with yeast.
12. Only take foods prepared fresh for each meal.

Common Cold

There are several practices which will greatly speed up recovery from this pernicious nuisance:
1. The first thing to remember with all diseases is that with the onset of symptoms, immediately lie down and change your nostril. If your left nostril is working, lie down on your left side until the right is thoroughly open; and vice versa. This procedure changes body chemistry by switching brain dominance from one hemisphere to another. If the nostril refuses to change, plug it with a cotton ball. Above all, never breathe through the mouth.
2. Start the day with the honey-pepper mixture

described under the Black Pepper section.

3. Following the black pepper, swallow, without chewing, one-half an average garlic clove with a glass of lukewarm water. This adds heat to the system.

4. Take tea made from water, one tablespoon of fenugreek seeds, seven black peppercorns, and one teaspoon of fresh, minced ginger. Boil in two cups of water until one cup remains. Black tea may be added, as may sugar. The boiled ingredients may be used two or three times. Take three or four times daily at most.

5. Never take sour foods when suffering from a cold, when weather is cold and damp, or after nightfall. Sour foods irritate the throat and increase coughing. Take no cold foods or liquids and drink as much lukewarm water as possible. Avoid eating radishes.

6. Sit facing a fire as much as possible. Fire has a great power to draw toxins from the body in the form of perspiration. The sweat of a sick person smells bad because it contains poisons which are being flushed from the system.

7. Keep the body well-covered from throat to thighs to conserve heat — wool clothing is best. Avoid all synthetic fabrics.

8. Take the red bottle sugar candy described in the section on Light and Medicine, at the end of this chapter.

9. Take twice daily a mixture of one-half teaspoon each: fresh ginger juice and honey.

10. Massage the chest region with mustard oil prepared in the following manner:

Boil two cloves of garlic in one-half cup mustard oil until the garlic completely burns. Remove the oil and cool.

Now apply a few drops of the oil to the navel, one drop in each nostril and a few drops in each ear.

If possible, this oil should be made in advance. Keep half in a red bottle and half in a blue bottle and keep both bottles in direct sunlight for 40 days. Use the oil from the red bottle for the nostrils and ears and blue bottle oil for the eyes.

11. Sleep with the head lower than the feet to increase the flow of blood to the head.

12. Do head stands as frequently as possible, but never during daylight hours. After the head stand, jump up and down three times to free the muscles and nerves, walk briskly for a few minutes and then lie down in the corpse position for twenty minutes.

13. One who is suffering from a cold should bathe in warm water. This practice prevents the draining of bodily heat necessary for fighting the disorder.

14. The old maxim "Feed a cold and starve a fever" holds true. A victim of cold suffers loss of energy, and needs as much food as possible to restore heat to the system. A fever, conversely, is excessive heat, and thus little food should be given — mainly liquids to flush the system.

15. To prevent colds, keep the feet covered and warm in cold weather and wet weather. Cover the throat region with a scarf, and the abdomen and pelvis should be kept warm. Before going out into cold weather, especially when wind is also present, plug the ears with small wads of cotton. By these simple procedures most colds can be prevented.

Constipation

The problem of constipation can be approached simultaneously on three fronts: general living principles, diet and medication. Because no two human systems are identical, everyone will have to find the combination best suited for himself. In general, all the daily living and dietary practices may be followed simultaneously. But only one medication should be pursued at any given time, and it is best to discontinue a medical practice after 40 days so that the system, now functioning properly, can become self-sufficient. The first rule in all cases is getting up before dawn.

General Practices:

1. Keep fresh water in a solid, unsoldered copper or silver pot about a foot from the crown of the head during sleep. Cover with a cheesecloth to keep out dust and lint. During sleep the brain expends considerable electrical energy in dreaming. Water and copper (or silver) are both conductors, and will catch and store much of this energy. Following the getting up rituals, drink the water before going to the bathroom to recapture this vital energy. This is a good lifetime practice, and should restore clean movements in a few days.

2. After drinking the water, take a long slow walk in the morning air. This starts the downward flow of gases essential to proper motion, as well as giving you fresh air and the tranquil beauty of the early morning.

3. Sit in the squatting (crouched) position as often as possible, keeping the feet flat on the ground. This opens the muscles of the pelvic region and also helps relaxation into the proper posture for defecation.

4. Never wear tight-fitting clothing or belts. These block the downward flow of gases, as well as disturbing the natural breath cycle.

5. Take regular tub baths in lukewarm water. Do not spend too much time in the tub, and do not allow the mind to wander. Never use warm water on the head.

6. Cut down or stop the use of tobacco. Smoking dries the system, impeding the passage of stools.

7. During sleep always lay on the left side — not

curled up, however. This practice keeps the right nostril open, the best nostril for digestion, as well as relieving pressure on the digestive tract — helping food to pass downward without obstruction.

8. Never sleep during the day or within three hours of taking food.

Dietary Practices:

1. Irregular eating habits may be the single greatest reason, besides sleeping past sunrise, for morning constipation. Hindu scriptures say that one who eats once a day never gets sick, one who eats twice, rarely. But he who eats often is seldom well... A few general principles to follow are:

   A. Never eat more than twice a day.

   B. Avoid all in-between-meal snacks.

   Frequent eating keeps the digestive system in a state of constant excitation, leaving no time for either rest or thorough digestion.

2. Fast one day a week, preferably the same weekday on which you were born. Drink only buttermilk, lemon-water with honey, or plain water during the fast day.

3. Eat only when the right nostril operates. Drink only when the left operates.

4. Drink plenty of water during the day — a gallon is recommended — to keep the system well moistened and free-flowing.

5. Avoid coffee and tea. Both dry the system and should be used as infrequently as possible. But, if you must take either, add a quarter teaspoon of butter per cup.

6. Never take tea or coffee within a half-hour of meals, before or after.

7. Hot spicy food draws water from the system, and should generally be avoided. Cereals (cracked wheat and oats especially) should be dietary staples. After

browning in a dry frying pan, add water and boil until thoroughly cooked; then add milk and sugar only when served.

8. Never drink milk which has been boiled for more than a few seconds. Milk which has been boiled twice, or boiled more than a few seconds, is very constipating. Fresh whole milk, on the other hand, helps prevent constipation.

9. Eat and drink only when sitting down and relaxed. Food taken when standing — or when tense or anxious — does not digest properly.

10. Following the morning meal, lay down on your left side for 20 minutes. This keeps your right nostril open and aids digestion.

11. Take a long, leisurely walk after the evening meal.

12. Never eat after sunset or within three hours of sleep. This gives food time to digest properly before sleep, when energies are drawn to the head during dreaming.

Medications:

Medicinal treatment should only be used when other approaches have met with failure.

1. *Malai:* Take two teaspoons of the skim which forms on hot milk. Heat milk to boiling point, then allow to simmer until enough *malai* collects on the surface. Take this with a dash of black pepper each night before retiring. This should restore clear motion in two days, prompt regularity in 15, after which it should be discontinued.

2. *Sat Isabgol:* This is an Indian remedy (fleaseed husk) available only from importers. Take one to two teaspoons in yogurt or water before retiring. Discontinue after 40 days.

3. Stewed prunes: Three to five prunes boiled 15 minutes or longer taken in the morning are a great aid to regularity. Figs may also be prepared

in the same fashion.

4. *Ajwain:* A mixture of ½ teaspoon each of oregano seed (*ajwain*) and baking soda with a dash of salt washed down with lukewarm water settles stomach distress which can lead to irregularity.

5. Enemas: A final recourse never to be done more than once a week.

Cough

Victims of severe coughing should avoid all milk and dairy products (which produce mucous) and citrus fruits (which irritate the throat), and radishes especially when bronchitis is present.

For severe cough due to colds, take a mixture of one tablespoon each of freshly squeezed onion or ginger juice.

Other remedies include:

1. Use red cardamom seeds when the throat feels irritated. Keep them in the mouth, chewing slowly and allowing the juice to slide down the throat. This relieves irritation and prevents unnecessary cough.

2. Make tea using licorice roots. Also, keep flakes of licorice root in your mouth and chew, sucking the juice. Spit out the pulp after all taste has vanished.

3. Sit near a fire as much as possible with the chest facing the flames.

4. Don't smoke.

5. Don't eat after sunset. Coughing troubles increase after sunset.

6. Sleep with the chest region higher than the feet.

7. Vomit each morning after defecation, using a pint or more of lukewarm salt water.

8. Keep a piece of black salt in the mouth, letting it dissolve slowly, swallowing the juice. This may be purchased at an Indian food store.

9. Boil a quart of goat's milk to which has been added

one-half teaspoon each of roasted turmeric and oregano seeds and an ounce of *jaggery* (*gur*, an unrefined sugar available from Indian food stores) until the mixture becomes one-fourth the original quantity. Divide into four equal parts and allow to cool. Take one dose after sunrise and the second after sunset. If trouble remains after two days, make another batch. *This medication is also a sure cure for whooping cough in infants.*

10. Drink only lukewarm water — avoid all cold drinks.
11. Avoid all alcoholic beverages.
12. Chew a fresh whole clove, swallowing the juice to open the nerves and make breathing smoother.

Cuts

Immediately after the cut has taken place one should press the tissue just above the injury so that blood does not flow out or air leave the nerves. Then pour sugar over the wound to stop blood flow.

Raw or brown sugar mixed with enough mustard oil to insure adhesion may be placed on an open wound, then covered with a bandage. A clean cloth soaked in fresh water, mustard oil, or coconut oil also works well. Alum powder sprinkled on a cut coagulates and stops the flow of blood.

Grind together equal parts of oregano seeds and *jaggery*. This is very useful when there is a sliver which cannot be removed easily with a needle. Just apply this mixture, and bandage. The splinter of sliver will work its way out overnight.

The beeswax ointment described in the section on Bedsores is useful for all open wounds.

Cysts

The following fomentation is a good cure for cysts, ganglions and other subcutaneous infections:

Wear the same pair of cotton or wool socks waking and sleeping — and without washing them — for 14 days. (This sounds terrible, doesn't it? but we assure you it works.) This means they should be worn at all times, save when bathing, meditating and eating. At the end of the two weeks put one sock aside for later use as needed. Fill the other sock with rock salt which has been heated on an open wood fire to the hottest tolerable temperature. Use about two ounces of salt.

Now apply the sock to the area over the cyst until the heat is gone. *Tantric* texts recommend repeating the sound "Vishnu" silently over and over, as long as the sock is on the skin. Do this each morning until the cyst disappears.

Wearing the socks for two weeks permeates the fibres with the salt produced by the body in perspiration. The heated salt in turn draws perspiration from the body into the sock, dissolving some of the salt inside. Salt water conducts heat and electricity better than any other medium, allowing them to reach beneath the skin directly to the site of the infection and greatly speeding the healing process.

The area may also be massaged with mustard oil to which a pinch of salt has been added, rubbing in a clockwise direction with the index finger of the right hand.

One may also use the cotton ball and oil fomentation described in the section on Bedsores.

Eyesight

In addition to cleansing the nostrils and regularly washing the eyes, there are other practices which will help correct faulty vision and prevent visual disorders for those with healthy eyes:

1. Meditate daily on a flame as described in the chapter on *Tratak*.
2. The soot of the *ghee* lamp, called *kajal*, may be

collected on a spoon held over the flame. Just rub a small amount on the inside of each lower eyelid, using the right ring finger. This can be done daily after meditation.

3. Use rosewater, mustard oil or honey in the eyes at least once daily. You may prefer to use honey and mustard oil after going to bed as they sting for several minutes.
4. Avoid using eyeglasses whenever possible to minimize dependence.
5. Walk barefoot on dewy grass in the morning.
6. Avoid getting steam in the eyes or using hot water on the head.
7. Massage the feet daily with mustard oil, especially the region between the big and second toes. Nerves ending here connect directly to the visual centre of the brain.
8. Never sit with the feet exposed to a fire.
9. Detailed, close work should be avoided at night, in poor lighting conditions and at the time of sunrise and sunset.

Eye Irritation

When the eyes become irritated due to overwork or the presence of foreign matter, first fill the mouth with cool water and then splash water of the same temperature into the open eyes while swishing water through the teeth. Splashing the eyes seven times seems to be the most effective practice.

If burning or irritation persists, a few drops of rosewater may be used in each eye. One drop of *ghee* (clarified butter) or honey in each eye is also a good cleanser. If you wish to keep rosewater ready for use as an eye medication (a good idea), store in a blue bottle in the refrigerator.

If toxic substances have burned the eyes, first rinse thoroughly as described above, then follow up with a rinse of tea which has been allowed to cool to room temperature. The eyes should then be covered with slices of raw potato until all traces of pain disappear. Potato slices draw the toxins out of the eyes and will turn brown as they work.

Another substance which draws poisons from the eyes may be made as follows: make a ball of wheat flour the size of a small plum and divide into two equal parts. Apply a few drops of *ghee* to each and flatten into disks large enough to completely cover the eyes. Now close the eyes, cover with dough and rest for 40 minutes.

Falls

If you fall down, immediately *jump* to your feet if there is no sign of a broken bone. This restores the flow of energy through the nerves and prevents shock and secondary reactions.

If the body has become bruised, superficially or deep, heat provides the most effective form of treatment. An electric hotpad is excellent and should be as hot as the victim can tolerate comfortably.

Mustard oil which has been heated to the point of sizzling and allowed to cool can be rubbed onto the affected area and is especially beneficial if a little bit of salt is first added to the oil.

If there is a painful bruise, a sprain or any sign of swelling, heat a half-tablespoon of turmeric in a half-cup of mustard oil with a pinch of salt and two garlic cloves. Heat on medium-high flame until both turmeric and garlic have charred completely. Strain the oil, allow to cool to a tolerable temperature and apply gently to injured area. This mixture stops pain and eliminates swelling.

An excellent ointment can be made from a third cup each of coconut, sesame and mustard oils. Mix on low heat and blend in one ounce of pure beeswax, a quarter-teaspoon of turmeric and a pinch of saffron.

After thoroughly blending, remove from heat, cool and apply to injured region. This is a fantastic ointment and should always be on hand for emergencies.

Fever

In cases of fever, the system is trying to purge itself of toxic substances which have infiltrated the tissues and circulatory system. All energies are needed to direct the body's cleansing mechanisms against the illness.

The old maxim "Feed a cold and starve a fever" should be made the general rule. Food demands the body divert energy from the site of the disease to the digestive organs, and with each meal the disease can reassert itself.

If the fever is prolonged, one may resort to the broths to provide nourishment for the system. In no cases should any dairy products be taken, nor any solid foods. Dairy products create an excess of mucous.

The patient of fever should drink as much warm water as possible, several gallons daily, to aid his system by continually flushing the tissues. Rest and relaxation are essential.

Generally, the fever should be allowed to run its course without recourse to antibiotics or similar medications. A fever is a cleansing device which can rid the system of poisons and waste matter accumulated over a period of months, even years.

However, prolonged or extremely high fevers can be injurious to the system, and in these cases a physician should be consulted.

For light fever the following can prove beneficial:
1. Almond oil, cold, on the top of the cranium either by soaking cotton strips or applying it on head and massaging gently, brings fever down and relieves the head of tension. Massage as described in the MASSAGE section is prohibited during fever.
2. Vinegar mixed with ice-cold water, which can be

applied the same way by putting cotton strips soaked in the abovementioned mixture on the top of the cranium, helps in lowering the temperature.

Gastritis

Gastritis is a collective term for a variety of closely linked disorders, all caused by the blockage of the downward flow of gases in the intestinal tract. Gases residing in the lower abdomen are responsible for forcing waste materials from the system — including urination, defecation, ejaculation, farting and the contractions which force the child from the womb in childbirth. *Yoga* physiology calls these gases *apana*.

Even chronic anxiety constricts the anal sphinctre, *apana* can no longer flow freely in a downward direction. As pressure builds up, the gas must move — and so begins to rise upward through the system. Instead of passing out as flatus, the *apana* forces its way upward into the stomach — where it is either retained or expelled as belching.

Because *apana* has come from the lower intestines, it is permeated with wastes discharged by the body into the excretory system — especially true if bowel movement has not occurred. These wastes are toxic chemicals, very destructive to the sensitive tissues of the higher tract and capable of producing a broad spectrum of disorders of the stomach, intestines, heart, respiratory system, throat, head and brain (including many forms of schizophrenia and epilepsy.)

Gastritis is a universal disease in meat-eating cultures, produced by the chronic tension which results from over-stimulation of the nervous system by the large quantities of adrenalin and related neurostimulants found in meat. Common symptoms include continual hunger which actually increases after eating a regular-sized meal, early morning constipation, frequent belching and hiccoughing, chronic hyperacidity, abdominal distention, ulcers, reflex esophagitis, etc.

TREATMENT: Gastritis can be approached on three basic fronts: lifestyle, diet and medication. The basic treatment for this and all other diseases is awakening well before sunrise. Late rising is a direct cause of chronically disturbed gases. No cure of *apana*-related disorders is possible without early rising.

Morning constipation has been discussed at length at the end of the chapter on Waking Up, and this aspect of the disease should be treated as outlined in that section. Regulating bowel movements is the key to the cure of gastritis — a prompt early morning movement discharges all bad gases.

The patient of gastritis should avoid all foods which produce excessive quantities of gas. A partial list includes: meat, eggs, fish, canned foods, prepared foods, leftovers, greasy and fried foods, milk which has been cooked long or boiled twice; raw nuts, large amounts of roasted nuts (any number over five), cabbage, cauliflower, lentils, legumes, rice, pickles, red and green peppers, fats and oils, cheese and curds, and large quantities of citrus juices. The use of ginger in cooking is very helpful as this spice kills gas when used properly. A pinch of asafoetida is also good in foods to kill gas — but overuse dries the system and makes matters worse.

Large quantities of coffee and tea are to be avoided. Under no circumstances should raw vegetables, raw nuts, raw seeds and raw fruits (especially apples) be taken. The only exceptions are coconut — especially the milk — and pineapple. All vegetables should be thoroughly boiled to insure easy digestion.

Permissible foods include squash, spinach which has been boiled with garlic, a small amount of fresh (not frozen) sweet peas, potatoes in small amounts, tomatoes (cooked), cucumbers which have been boiled as a vegetable, cereals (especially cracked wheat, cream of wheat and rolled oats — all browned in a hot, dry frying pan before boiling and never boiled in milk).

papaya, pomegranate, lemon juice in water and mu and chamomile teas.

Two foods may be cooked in milk: papaya and bottle squash. Both should be peeled and grated before cooking. Raw sugar may be added to the papaya. After cooking either one, add a pinch of crushed red cardamom seeds before serving.

To promote proper digestion, a glass of lemon water may be taken as needed between 30 minutes and an hour after meals. Juice one lemon in a glass of lukewarm water, making sure no seeds remain in the glass. Add a pinch of black salt and drink.

The gelatinous substance from the inside of aloevera (aloe) leaves is a great medicine for gastritis. The contents of one leaf, sprinkled lightly with freshly ground black pepper, should be taken daily before any other food or drink is introduced into the system.

Plain lemon juice and water is an excellent early morning drink when conditions are aggravated, but should not be made a regular medication and should never be taken when there is any sign of hyperacidity. If acidity is present, add a teaspoon of baking soda to the drink before taking.

One practice which may be carried out daily is to take one-half of an average garlic clove, swallowed without chewing with a glass of lukewarm water. Done each morning before breakfast for 40 days, this is a great help in cases of chronic gastritis.

As an emergency measure when gases are rising at any time, mix together on a piece of paper the size of a matchbook cover a half-teaspoon each of baking soda and oregano seeds (*ajwain*) and sprinkle with a dash or two of salt. Tilt the head back and swallow the mixture dry, then wash down with a glass of lukewarm water. This immediately kills gases.

As a general practice, follow the steps outlined for morning constipation and NEVER EAT, MEDITATE OR ENGAGE IN STRENUOUS PHYSICAL

ACTIVITIES BEFORE MORNING BOWEL MOVE-MENT. Otherwise the flow of gases will be severely disturbed and a whole host of ailments may result.

A General Tonic

From a handful of small beans daily, one can make a tonic which provides the body with iron in its most useful form — a potent and natural medication for fighting anemia and blood deficiencies, and for providing growing systems with a vital natural chemical.

All one needs is *channa dal* (a small, brown bean available at Indian import stores and from Rams Head) which is whole (not split or peeled). Only the whole grains are suitable for sprouting, the secret of this tonic.

For a child, take 10 beans and place in a cast iron pot with enough water to cover. Now cover the pan with a strainer or cheesecloth, making sure both air and light can reach the beans. Within a day, the beans should begin to sprout (though it may take more time depending on temperature and pressure). Allow the young shoots to grow until they attain the length of a fingernail.

Now take the water in which the sprouts have grown and pour into a glass. Drink, after adding honey or raw sugar and rosewater to taste. Then take the raw, fresh sprouts and chew slowly until well-masticated (to insure easy digestion) before swallowing.

For an adult, one should take a level handful of beans for sprouting, though older persons should take the same number of sprouts as a child — 10.

This tonic works from age four to the grave and is especially powerful to correct food deficiencies. It works as well to stimulate brain tissues, lungs and the whole vascular system. It is especially useful for newly-weds who wish to keep their level of energy up.

For best results, prepare regularly and take every morning, early enough in the day so that the system has time to digest the sprouts.

Headache

At the first sign of a headache, immediately note which nostril is working — then lie down on the same side to change your breath. This method will head off the worst of migraines. If some symptoms still persist, tie a tourniquet around the elbow on the same side of the body as the head pain and keep it on until the pain vanishes.

If one ignores the first warning signs and the headache develops, there are several measures which can be taken:

1. Apply a paste of freshly ground clay to the forehead. Let dry completely, then rub off by hand and wash. A paste made from the ground hulls of red cardamom may be used in the same fashion.
2. Equally good, if not better, is a paste made from freshly ground sandalwood (grind a piece of sandalwood on a slightly rough stone with a few drops of water until a thick paste is formed. Now add a pinch each of saffron and camphor and grind until thoroughly blended. Apply as above.)
3. If not suffering from symptoms of a cold, drink a teaspoon of honey in a glass of warm water, or
4. Fill the stomach completely with water, or
5. Massage forehead, temples, neck and shoulder muscles using the procedures outlined in the chapter on Massage. Be sure to use a little organic oil on the hands to prevent chafing and burning.
6. If before sunrise or after sunset and the stomach is empty, do a head stand. This increases blood flow in the head and stops most forms of headache.

Heart Ailments

In addition to adopting the practices for daily life outlined elsewhere in this work, patients of heart ailments should adopt the basic diet for a gastritis patients outlined earlier in this section. The practice of taking half of a medium garlic clove swallowed whole with warm water early each morning is especially helpful. Clear, bowel movements are also necessary.

Never suppress any natural functions, especially defecation, farting, belching, coughing and sneezing. Stopping these natural processes allows disturbed gases to rise and affect the heart.

To the extent possible, avoid all injected medications. That part not assimilated by the body tends to congeal on the arterial walls near the heart — which can seriously aggravate cardiac disorders.

Avoid anxiety, grief, fear and sexual arousal. These emotional states cause an imbalance of blood chemistry which weakens the heart.

Only speak the truth. The act of telling a lie quickens the heartbeat and creates fear. Similarly, one should avoid all actions which he feels are immoral, or which produce guilt.

Don't read newspapers, news magazines or listen to radio or television newscasts. Only "exciting" items, especially disasters, catastrophes and suspense, make the news. All have a tendency to cause arousal and quicken the heart.

Avoid sex. In lovemaking the speed of the heart increases dramatically, and can induce heart attacks (as we have all heard.)

Basically, patients of heart ailments should never allow their peace of mind to be disturbed — even at the cost of all personal wealth.

Helpful practices for heart patients include:

1. Walk barefoot in fresh green grass as often as possible. This is a very soothing experience, excellent for calming the nerves.

2. Use flowers and keep them around as much as possible. Flowers provide soothing visual images and the odour of flowers has a very helpful chemical effect on the nervous system and heart. Visit gardens as often as possible.

3. Drink water from a silver pot. Silver ions enter the water and strengthen the system.
4. Stop tobacco, coffee and tea. Instead drink pure glucose, one teaspoon to a glass of lukewarm water. Use iron and calcium in organic form.
5. Always avoid sudden changes in temperature, including baths either too hot or too cold. In cold weather be sure to keep the region from chin to thighs well covered. NEVER TAKE A SAUNA BATH.
6. Take 2-3 sheets of silver paper (available from Indian import stores) with fresh fruit (papaya is best) early in the morning.

Insomnia

For those experiencing difficulties in sleeping, several practices are commonly employed by Indian healers:
1. Eat a good meal shortly before sunset, followed two hours later by a bath in lukewarm water. The patient should now go to bed, preferably listening to either drone instruments or the sound of rustling leaves.
2. The milk of a nursing mother brings immediate sleep when one drop is placed in each of the subject's nostrils.
3. Rinse the eyes with rosewater, then add a drop of *ghee* (clarified butter) to each eye. Keep eyes closed and sleep.
4. Comb the hair before retiring.
5. Massage the feet, calves, nape of neck and shoulders.
6. If married, engage in sex.

The remedies just cited are for periodic insomnia. If the condition is chronic, one then knows that the brain cells are receiving insufficient fluid and the nervous system is afflicted by a superabundance of heat. This condition occurs frequently in the more acute phases of schizophrenia.

In chronic cases of insomnia, the sulfur medication described in the SCHIZOPHRENIA section should be given immediately. Additionally, two to three gallons of lukewarm water should be consumed daily, and sandalwood paste liberally applied to forehead, earlobes, crown of head, nipples and navel. These practices, when combined, will draw out excess heat and restore systemic balance.

Jaundice

Eliminate all high-protein foods from the diet immediately, and begin taking as much starch as possible. Under no circumstances eat meat, fish or eggs. Cheeses should be eliminated as well.

A tablespoon of pure glucose (not table sugar, which is to be avoided at all costs) added to a glass of lukewarm water and mixed with the juice of a fresh lemon provides a drink which is especially beneficial to the liver and kidneys. This should be taken from 16 to 30 times daily as long as symptoms persist. Lemon flushes excess bile from the system.

Eat radishes as often as possible. This food helps purify the system of toxins. It is a good idea to start the day with a half-cup of fresh radish juice and a teaspoon of honey. Another good drink is fresh sugarcane juice. Molasses and water is also helpful.

Kidney Ailments

For disturbances of the kidneys and urinary system, the butter-milk drink should be taken at least three times daily: once in the morning, a second glass in the early afternoon and the third with the evening meal. This stimulates the healing process and cures the depression and pessimism often caused by kidney disorders — including those attributable to excessive use of alcohol.

Radishes are excellent for kidney disorders. They are

a powerful diuretic which stimulate the flow of urine and release of toxins from the body.

Tea, coffee and other stimulating drinks should be eliminated from the diet, and no juices with a high sugar content should be used. Drink as much water as possible to keep the flow of poisons from the body as strong as possible. Vinegar and onions, prepared in salads and served with meals, are very helpful.

Muscular Aches, Sprains and Bruises

For spastic aches and pains due to sprains or bruises apply the following poultice:

Boil together one-half cup of mustard oil, one tablespoon of turmeric, one-eighth teaspoon of calcium hydroxide and a pinch of table salt. The mixture will first turn red, then brown. Once browned, remove from heat and soak a clean cloth in the solution. Allow the cloth to cool to a tolerable temperature, apply to skin over the injured area and allow to stand for two to three hours, breathing through the left nostril as long as the medication rests on the body.

Don't use this poultice more than twice on any given injury or damage can result to the sensitive tissues of the skin.

A variation on this same solution also works well: prepare all ingredients as above, except salt, and with the addition of two cloves of garlic. Cook until garlic has completely burned. Remove from heat and strain into glass or ceramic container. Use the oil for massaging the injured area, then cover with a clean, dry cloth and relax for one or two hours.

If neither of the above formulas can be made, boil ordinary straw in water, strain and apply the straw to the surface of the injured area once it has cooled to a tolerable temperature.

Piles

Piles are small fleshy masses appearing at the mouth of the anal passage, characterized by pain, itching, burning and often bleeding. In the case of bleeding piles, blood should be allowed to drain out completely before the application of any medicine (otherwise impure blood will be trapped inside the sore, allowing infection to develop and spread). General practices for patients of this common disorder include:

1. Don't sit for a prolonged period on hard seats. A cotton-filled pillow, preferably made of deerskin and covered with a white cloth, works best.
2. Never ignore the natural urges for defecation, urination, coughing, sneezing, farting or belching.
3. Never sit for a long time on the toilet seat. Use the squatting posture for defecation.
4. Avoid frequent eating, cutting food intake to one or at the most two meals daily — and eliminating all snacks.
5. Eat food which contains bulk and is easily digested. Wheat, barley and oat cereals are excellent, with a little milk added after cooking. Squash and amaranthus which have been peeled and well boiled are also good.
6. Avoid greasy foods, fried foods, anything which has been frozen or is served cold directly from the refrigerator. Eliminate from the diet all beef, fish, pork, dried meat, curds, cheeses, sesame, canned food and any foods cooked more than four hours previously.
7. Take one or two glasses daily of the buttermilk mixture.
8. Follow the general practices outlined in the section on constipation at the end of the first chapter.
9. Take a ball of beeswax about the size of a pencil eraser each morning for 40 days. Chew thoroughly

and swallow, washing it down with warm — *not hot* — milk.

Poisoning

In cases of oral poisoning, boil a cup or more of wheatgerm in a large pot of water until the water becomes thoroughly red. Strain out the germ and pour the water into as many glasses as necessary. To each glass add a tablespoon of *ghee* and a teaspoon of salt. Swallow one or two glasses immediately. Vomiting will follow almost at once. Repeat this procedure five or six times, until the stomach has been thoroughly purged.

Vomiting empties the stomach of toxic contents, and the chemicals of the wheatgerm and *ghee* purify the system by drawing out and neutralizing toxins.

Taken immediately, milk is a very beneficial antidote for many varieties of poisoning. The most harmful agents in the toxin attack the milk, diminishing their effect on the human system.

Poison Ivy, Poison Oak

For poison ivy, poison oak and similar painful irritations of the outermost layer of the skin, one should avoid all heat-producing foods, salt, sugar, and potatoes.

A most effective medicine can be made from plain yogurt and a handful of copper pennies. Place 20 copper pennies in a bowl with a half-cup of yogurt. Stir to mix thoroughly and allow to stand. Within minutes the yogurt will begin to turn blue as the coins give off copper sulphate. Once the yogurt has turned a medium shade of blue, apply to the affected skin. There will be a minute of moderately sharp pain as the mixture draws the heat out of the rash. Allow to dry and rub off.

Now massage into the skin *ghee* which has been treated as follows:

Take three tablespoons of clarified butter in a cereal

bowl, add crushed ice or ice cubes along with enough cold water to cover. Whip thoroughly with the fingers and change water after the *ghee* begins to turn lighter in colour.

Use no more ice cubes, but continue whipping with cool water, changing frequently, until 108 complete revolutions of the hand have been made. By this time the *ghee* will have lost all yellow colouring and have become a white, light, spongy substance. This *ghee* is now an excellent ointment for rubbing onto rashes caused by poison ivy or oak, itches, and other persistent skin infections where there is redness. Under no circumstance should *ghee* prepared in this fashion be taken orally or used in the eyes, as it has become a poison.

Until the redness vanishes, one should avoid wetting the infected area of the skin. Before bathing, mustard oil may be applied as a coating over the affected area, or the ointment described at the end of the section on FALLS may be applied before taking a bath.

Following the bath, an application of copper-yogurt followed by *ghee* is helpful. This treatment may be repeated once or twice daily until the redness vanishes.

Schizophrenia

Not a single disorder, but a set of symptoms resulting from a severe disturbance of the bodily elements, schizophrenia can be described as a disbalance in energy which produces a lack of ability to concentrate, extreme anxiety and bizarre (aberrative) behaviours.

In all cases of extreme emotional disturbance, one should first ensure a regular bowel movement each morning. In virtually all cases of schizophrenia there is retention of the feces, often for several days at a time. See specific remedies for constipation.

Many times the schizophrenic patient will be found to be suffering from acute forms of gastritis, and adoption of the treatment for this ailment outlined earlier in this section is advisable.

Daily application of sandal paste to the back of the head (in a ring shape), earlobes, throat, nipples and navel helps alleviate nervous tension and break compulsive behaviour patterns. Make the paste by grinding a block of sandalwood on a slightly rough stone, using a few drops of water. Add a pinch each of saffron and camphor and continue grinding. Apply as a thick paste and lie down in the corpse posture for 30 minutes, breathing deeply and slowly through the left nostril in a 1-4-2 cycle (inhale for one beat, retain the air for four and exhale for two). Do this each morning until conditions improve.

Another helpful medication which relieves the excessive heat found in the brain of schizophrenics can be made by keeping mustard oil in a blue bottle and exposing it to direct sunlight for 15-40 days. Massage a small amount daily into the top of the head. Coconut oil to which a few drops of pure sandalwood oil (not essence) has been added will also work.

Patients should avoid all disturbing, fast-paced music and listen instead to the soothing sounds of drone instruments, preferably the *tamboura*. Salt and all drying substances should be eliminated from the diet. Coffee, tea and tobacco are injurious. Similarly, mind-altering drugs can greatly aggravate the schizophrenic symptoms and should be avoided at all times.

Bathing in cool water, a few degrees below room temperature, or a fresh water creek or spring is also very beneficial. But the schizophrenic patient should under no circumstances bathe in salt water, which dries the system.

Malai, a skim from milk which has been allowed to simmer for an hour or more, is of great help in relieving internal dryness. Take two teaspoons with a pinch of sugar and freshly ground red cardamom each evening before bed. But under no circumstances drink the milk from which *malai* has been prepared — it produces dryness and constipation.

Synchronizing with the natural cycles of sun and moon is of primary importance. The first two steps should be regularity in arising before dawn and synchronizing the nostrils with the moon cycle for the first three days following the darkest and full moon nights.

Schizophrenia is a disease of cycles: the patient will be found to be more violence-prone during the ascending moon cycle, more depressed in the descending cycle.

The system of the schizophrenic will be found to have a diminished sulphur content. This can be corrected by using the following medication:

Melt one ounce of organic sulphur over a wood fare, but do not allow to burn. Dip the sulfur into a pot of milk which has a cheesecloth lining the bottom. When the sulphur has cooled, pull up the cheesecloth to remove the congealed sulphur. Reheat and repeat the process. This should be done exactly 108 times, and the milk in the pot changed after each 15 dippings.

Now the molecular structure of the sulphur has changed to become a form readily assimilated by the system. One dose taken each morning for 40 days will restore normal moistness to the system. Calculate the dose as follows: for ages five through eight, two pieces; nine through sixteen, three pieces; and four pieces for an adult.

Sulphur prepared in this fashion provides an excellent remedy for all diseases connected with system dryness, including excema, some cases of leprosy and the dryness caused by retention of feces.

Again, schizophrenia is not a single disease, and so it is impossible to outline a specific course of treatment without considering the variations in individual body chemistry. The procedures outlined here are designed to alleviate the more commonly associated complaints.

Skin Diseases

The vast majority of skin diseases can be directly attributed to impurities of the blood. Leucoderma, lichen, boils, acne, rash, itch and obnoxious body odours all are results of chemical imbalances of the circulatory system.

The chick pea flour and mustard oil (*ubtan*) application described in the chapter on Massage is most beneficial for all skin disorders.

One who suffers from or is easily susceptible to skin ailments should avoid the use of intoxicants, salt, sesame oil, potatoes, green vegetables, curd, vinegar and all foul-smelling foods.

Day sleep, over-eating, frequent eating and eating after sunset should always be avoided, as should anger, prolonged exposure to sun, working to the point of fatigue and basking before a fire.

Drinking large quantities of room temperature water helps purify the system by flushing out toxins. One should drink at least a gallon daily.

Daily application of a thin clay paste also helps in cases of acne, rash, itch, ichthyosis and similar skin ailments by drawing out and absorbing poisons. Apply paste, allow to dry (in the sun if possible), rub off with fingers and rinse.

For troublesome pimples and sties on the eyelids, apply freshly ground whole cloves. This both relieves pain and heals the infection.

Sore Throat

When the throat becomes sore from infection, smoking or system dryness, one may gargle with alum powder to alleviate immediate symptoms. Mix one teaspoon in a glass of lukewarm water and gargle. If alum is not available, a tablespoon of salt is also good.

When suffering from sore throat, all sour foods should

be avoided, as they will cause further irritation. This includes yogurt, citric juices and all fruits. Hot foods, cold foods and tobacco also create further irritation.

The honey-pepper mixture described in the BLACK PEPPER section will help in mild cases, though it should not be used when the throat tissues are extremely sensitive. Sucking on a fresh clove will help in these cases, for the juice of the clove is a mild anesthetic.

Toothache

To kill both the pain and infection of toothache, chew a clove slowly — allowing the juice to penetrate the affected region. To fight off the infection, eat red peppers and orange juice (fresh); both contain high amounts of vitamin C. Eat as much ginger as possible, especially in the winter.

The teeth should always be brushed twice daily. To keep teeth strong and prevent future trouble, always clench the jaws together as tightly as possible during urination and defecation.

Treatment by Light

The body is a temple of consciousness built of five basic elements, the *tattwas*. The proportion of elements varies from individual to individual, and within the individual from moment to moment. This ebb and flow of elements is in a natural process.

Disease is a state resulting from prolonged imbalance in the interplay of earth, water, fire, air — and *Akash*.

We have already discussed how these elements underlie the Ayurvedic system, as well as the understanding of diet — and its regulation. The same principles of *vayu* (wind), *pitta* (bile), and *kapha* (mucous) are at work in the practice of using light to treat physical and emotional disturbances.

Each element vibrates within a frequency range

corresponding to the harmonies of visible light spectrum. Colours are light energy in different wave lengths, they may stimulate or inhibit growth and development of an organism. Light influences the hormone discharge, hemoglobin formation, Thyroid activity, and liver's ability to detoxify foreign substances from the body chemistry. The entire segment of sympathic nervous system is influenced by the alternation of light and darkness. The study of impact of light on hypothalemic, pituitary, pineal — and adrenal mechanism which underlines the hormone rhythm, provides a clue to the awareness in birds and other animals which they exhibit by migrating at a right time. Light also effects the gonads, in total darkness gonads shrink to about a quarter of their normal size — and fertility is significantly reduced. It suggests that light can play an important role in the sexual behaviour and influence psyche by influencing neuroendoerine system. Utilising colours with the understanding of these harmonic correspondences provides a way to stimulate the restoration of proper balance, thus healing disorders of mind and body.

By exposing any substance to light of different colours, different responses will be noted. Some colours are hot, others cold. And prolonged exposure to light of one Colour can alter the elemental balance of the substance. These substances then can be used internally and externally to attain proper balance in body chemistry. These substances used to prepare medicines are

1. Water
2. Fruit Juices
3. Rock sugar candy
4. Oils.

Colours can be obtained directly by filtering sunlight through a coloured glass, or by using prolonged use of coloured lights. Sunlight however is the best — and coloured glass should be a piece of glass which has been given colour when it is made. Application of colour on glass to make it colourful is not as effective — as a piece of coloured glass. Use of coloured paper around white bottles also helps in obtaining a desired colour from sunlight. The paper used for this purpose is thin — and allows sunlight to permeate through it.

Ganges water, rain water or snow water left in coloured glass bottles in direct sunlight absorb energy in a few hours (as little as four), reaching peak of saturation in three days in India — and four days in countries where sunlight is not so powerful. This water is taken orally.

Fruit juices absorb energy even quicker and one hour exposure to brilliant sun light makes them potent with healing power obtained from the coloured light.

Water prepared in coloured bottles cannot be kept for a very long time — and fruit juices should never be stored for a long time. Water should be consumed within three days and fruit juices within an hour. Rock sugar candy can however be preserved for a longer period — and once they have been exposed to sunlight for a period of 40 days they can be used as long as they are rightly stored in cool and dry places. Rock sugar candy kept in coloured bottles for a period of 21 days absorbs enough energy for use as a healing agent. Small pieces of rock sugar candy should be taken orally and allowed to dissolve in mouth. By this process the medicine present in the rock sugar candy is assimilated into the blood vascular system by tiny capillaries present in the mouth.

Oils prepared in coloured bottles by direct exposure to sunlight are valuable because they can be easily preserved — and used for massaging the sick part of the body. Light (filtered through coloured glasses), water prepared in coloured bottles, juices — rock sugar candy — and oil may be used singly or in combination.

The basic colours used in preparing the medicine are: red, yellow, light orange, light blue, dark blue and green.

RED: Hot in nature, vitalizes all living matter — is positive magnetic vibration, serves as a wonderful healing agent in diseases of blood — and circulatory system, debility and depression, dysentery, pneumonia, joint pain, swellings caused by colds — and in driving poisons out from the body, plague boils, carbuncle, impotence, paralysis, serophia, tumors of all kinds — and all kinds of bone tuberculosis.

Red stimulates the arterial system and increases the amount of hemoglobin — and improves the circulation by raising body temperature. Red causes reaction to occur in release of adrenaline.

Because red colour is hot it beneficial to produce life in dead numb organs. Weakness, anemia and pessimism, dullness generally produced by lack of enthusiasm and inspiration. It is like a boon to old people, they regain their energy by regular use of water or juices prepared in red colour bottles after their morning — and evening meals. Red colour is also helpful in menstrual troubles, pain in waist region. Pain during or after menstruation, delay in period, irregularity of period. Exposure to red light and oral use of water prepared in red colour bottle is specially helpful to fat people because it reduces fat. While spots of leucoderma could be cured in primary stages by water charged with red colour. Red light exposed on white spot helps the de-coloured pigments to absorb colour. Red increases the amount of red blood corpuscles. It also can cure Hydroseal and filaria.

Water from red bottle, juices from red bottle or rock sugar candy increase energy — and stimulate the circulatory system — and can cause excitement, restlessness, anxiety, arrogance, irritability anger — and reasoning faculty. It should therefore be used carefully in lesser quantities — and should only be used after food and not on an empty stomach.

Use of red colour water on children below fifteen years of age is harmful. They should be given orange colour water if red is required by the system.

To get better results and quick recovery it is necessary to purify the organism by fasting on lemon water, water purification — sweating etc. This is the responsibility of the healer to see which method of purification will be most effective on his/her patient. *Oral use of medicine as well as using coloured light, massage of the afflicted areas — and a combination of proper diet bring quick recovery.*

ORANGE: Orange is also a hot colour in nature, although milder than red. It is good for ridding the stomach of mild poisons; it influences the digestive system and aids assimilation. Orange builds up energy in the body, cures disorders of the spleen, kidney disorders, bronchitis, congestion in the chest region and chronic asthma, venous debility, phlegmatic fevers, gout, wet cough and chronic rheumatism. The colour orange is especially remarkable in curing inflation of the kidneys, of kidney stones, prolapses, causation of menstruation, mental debility, pessimism, epilepsy and cholera.

Orange has a warming effect and is non-electrical and cheering. This colour is more suited to males than to females. It is especially beneficial for patients who suffer from chronic indigestion. The colour orange can safely be given to patients of all age groups. It cleans the upper and lower digestive tract, takes out deposited waste material from the stomach, and also from the intestines. It is slow in action and should therefore be used regularly for a longer period. After using it regularly for about three or four days one can feel the vitalising effect of the orange colour. It is a good colour to give as a tonic to weak patients.

The colour orange has a stimulating effect; someone using the orange colour should watch himself to see if one is getting overstimulated. Orange has a stimulating effect on goads and one could experience more sensual feelings or irritation. It is good to reduce the dosage when one experiences an overstimulation.

Orange take orally as water from an orange bottle, as juice from an orange bottle, or in the form of rock sugar candy will clean the stomach and intestines, and root out indigestion. Patients using orange orally should watch their stools and reduce the dosage if they find their stools getting thin.

For skin diseases, rashes, leprosy, leucoderma, the orange colour should be used orally and the patient should be advised to eat bread made from chickpeaflour, or garbanzobeanflour with a little butter. This bread is very healthy and useful if it is eaten when still fresh and warm. For removing kidney stone orange should be used in many ways: (1) orally, (2) by orange light in the afflicted area, (3) massage of the kidney region with oil from an orange bottle. These treatments will help dissolving the stone and flushing it out as small sand particles with the urine. The patient should avoid the use of milk, yoghurt, cheese, rice, sour things, including fruits, spinach and red chili.

The orange colour can cure heart burns, pain in the stomach, hysteria distaste, sour taste in the mouth, burps and sexual fever known as *Kama-Jwar* in Ayurvedic terminology.

YELLOW: Yellow is the most luminous and bright one of all colours. It has positive magnetic vibrations with a powerful effect on the nervous system. Yellow effects the brain directly and therefore is an important Colour for therapists who are working with patients of nervous diseases and mental illnesses.

Yellow is a ceremonial colour in India. Hindus wear a yellow dress while performing religious rites. And yellow is used by Brahmcharis (celebrates and students), by Buddhist monks and by monks of the Vaishnava order.

The yellow colour has affinity with the liver and the intestines, as this colour is found in bile (*pitta*). It is *pitta* that supplies a healthy glow to the skin, and while *pitta* is aggravated the colour of the skin and the eyes become yellow. Yellow thus also has a relationship with the skin, and has a healing effect on the skin.

Yellow stimulates mental faculties helping in creating

thoughts. Also it helps visualisation. Hindus and especially tantriks practice *tratak* on a ghee lamp flame which is luminous yellow. The yellow colour arouses optimism, makes one cheerful and provides a balanced outlook on life.

Yellow also is the colour of *vayu* (wind). *Vayu* works with the nervous system and disturbed *vayu* (apana) creates diseases of the nervous system and mental illnesses. The yellow colour therefore works with the two doshas *vayu* and *pitta*. Yellow therefore works with the skin, the digestive system, the organs of the abdominal region and the nervous system. It destroys germs, cures liver troubles, diabetes, bleeding piles and leprosy. Its nonstringent and alkaline effect strengthens the blood and the nervous system and cures dyspepsia when used orally. Also oil from a yellow bottle is used for massage on the abdominal region, but this should only be used for dyspepsia in which there is an increase of blue indicated by stoutness, which is caused by lack of exercise, or poor circulation. In this kind of dyspepsia fat increases, because of the increase of blue. The other kind of dyspepsia is the one in which there is an increase in the red; the patient becomes thin, has irritation in the stomach, hot hands, a hot head, and a feeling of heat. Massage with oil from an indigo bottle helps in this kind of dyspepsia and the patient should be given indigo coloured light on the abdominal region for a short period of time, along with the oral use of water, rock sugar candy, or juices from the indigo bottle. Patients of melancholy can be benefitted by the use of yellow, but patients who feel lonely should be kept away from the yellow colour.

During a treatment the therapist should watch the patient's skin colour, the colour of the eyes and the Colour of the nails carefully. If there is excess of yellow, then green should be used to create a balance.

The yellow colour can be used for asthma, inflammation of the lungs, bronchitis, liver congestion, mucous congestion, inflammation of the eyes, gas in the stomach, jaundice, constipation, indigestion, acidity, stiffness, amoebic dysentery, increasing fat, shaking or trembling of organs or of the whole body, spleen epilepsy, loss of speech, indigestion during pregnancy, delay in delivery, palpitation of the heart, and yellow can help mothers suffering from lack of milk in the breasts.

The colour yellow is good for infants.

GREEN: Green is a cool, refreshing and soothing colour. It is a mixture of hot yellow and cold blue. This combination provides green neutrality; it is neither heating, nor stringent, neither acidic, nor alkaline. The colour green provides a balance, and it has been observed that patients in mental hospitals like the green colour. Green provides an escape from anxiety. It has a resting and invigorating effect on the blood chemistry and a soothing effect on all the organs in general. Because of its cooling effect it works on eczema, sty, enlargement of the testicles, or burning sensation in the testicles, a wet vagina, a burning sensation in the intestines, abbesses in ears or breasts, ulcers (peptic or of intestines), hernia, tuberculosis of intestines, amoebic dysentery, blood dysentery, mucous in stools, colitis, syphilis, infections, black spots, bleeding from cuts, skin rashes, itchings, throat cancer, worms, blood in urine, gonorrhea, gum boils, urinary trouble during pregnancy, bleeding piles, blockage in the urinary tract, pain and burning during menstruation or overbleeding, red nose, ailments of the nose, stomach cancer, cracking of the walls of the female sex organs, wounds on the nipples after delivery, boils after delivery, itching in the ears, pain in the teeth, sinus trouble, deafness.

The colour green can be safely given orally and in combination with a light treatment and massage.

All non acidic or alkaline neutral foods should/ be given to patients during the use of the green colour.

Colour and Emotion

Exposure to light of different colours from filtered sun lamps in the 40 or so minutes before dawn helps create specific emotional frequencies in the human system. The body should be completely exposed to the light. Lie naked in the corpse position with eyes centred on the mid-brow region with lids open just enough to allow the colour to be perceived.

RED: Concentration on red stimulates frequencies useful for short, hard-term jobs to raise money. This colour also relieves digestive disorders and helps cure constipation.

ORANGE: increases sexual stamina.

BLUE: induces tranquillity, bringing one out of authoritarian ego trips.

GREEN OR GRAY: To resolve deep-seated emotional problems.

Wearing clothing of the same colour also produces the desired effects, though to a lesser degree. For example, wearing blue frequently can lead to constipation. Blue reduces heat in the system, which lowers digestive capacity. Children who wear blue frequently in childhood often develop digestive ailments later in life, while children who wear red eat much and can digest anything.

Pregnancy and Infant Care

Pregnancy is nothing to fear. Life's oldest miracle, the preservation of being, fulfils the deepest biological and psychic needs of the human organism.

Indian folk medicine offers some specific advice for expectant mothers. This can be broken down into biological functions, attitudes, and things to avoid.

Diet: The mother's diet is of critical importance during the nine months of pregnancy. From the food she consumes come the chemicals which will make up the body of her child. A strict vegetarian diet is, of course, the first fundamental rule to follow.

The blood of the mother is the sole source of nourishment for the child and so should be kept pure and healthy — rich in iron, oxygen, phosphorous and sugar. Sweet foods are very helpful.

Almond juices, extracted by the system from almond paste, provide a great source of nourishment for the development of the child's brain. Grind daily ten raw almonds which have soaked in room temperature water overnight into a paste on a slightly rough stone with a few drops of water and eat, saying "Vishnu." A child so nurtured during pregnancy develops an infallible memory.

And as almonds aid development of the brain, organic calcium facilitates development of eyes and skeletal system, so milk and yogurt should be taken.

The colour of the body is dependent on the amount of iron in the mother's bloodstream. Iron is essential — though in moderation. Raisins, figs, prunes, seeds, nuts (cashews, pistachios) are useful sources of this important mineral. Foods from this group should be consumed daily — though in small quantity (otherwise the child will become fat and hard to deliver).

While the sense organs of the child as well as the character of mind, intellect and memory are determined largely by past life *karmas*, their fullest possible development depends on consuming the right kinds of food in the right amounts. A mother should take part of the food her appetite demands, but not fill herself completely.

Similarly, an expectant mother should consume only food prepared fresh each day. Dry or old food should never be consumed. Instead, only palatable food cooked that day should be eaten.

BODY MOVEMENT: Because the bones and tissues of the developing fetus are delicate and easily damaged, a mother should take great care in the movement of her body.

She should not remain seated in one posture for too long a time. After each half hour she should arise, move about for a few minutes, then lie down and rest for a few minutes more.

Climbing of stairs is to be avoided because of the strain placed on the already expanded abdominal muscles. Similarly, repeated bending as well as sitting in difficult postures are to be avoided.

The mother should spend as much time as possible in the house, not roaming outside. (Similarly, frequent trips by car are to be abandoned.)

NATURAL FUNCTIONS: The expectant mother should pay attention to her bodily signals and take care of natural bodily functions as soon as she becomes aware of the need to do so.

The first rule concerns sleep. One should never sleep during the day — always be up before sunrise and remain conscious during the daylight hours. Sleep-fasts are to be avoided. Some sleep is necessary each night during the length of the term.

Under all circumstances she should go to the bathroom, sneeze, belch or pass gas whenever the urges are expereienced. Otherwise her gases will become disturbed, affecting the development and temperament of the child.

ATTITUDES TO ADOPT: The mother's feeling state is synchronous with the state of her body chemistry. Therefore, she must remain observant of her own feelings and, if necessary, change them.

Negative emotions affect not only her own feelings, but the body chemistry of the child she is carrying.

She should never be sad or worried. Why be sad when a new life is coming into the world? And why be worried? Whatever is God's will happens, despite all the worrying in the world. Similarly she should not be afraid — for what is there to fear? And so too for anger.

Instead, she should always be happy, dressing well

and devoting her thought to God and the miracle taking place within her body.

To help maintain these attitudes she should avoid all obnoxious and annoying people (including those who are angry, sad, worried, violent and quarrelsome). She should also avoid people with marked or obvious deformities, lest her impressions register on the infant.

People in this category include those who are deaf and dumb, blind, lame or marked by deformed limbs and features.

THINGS TO AVOID: This is a general category of actions and things the mother can avoid to ease pregnancy and delivery:

— Any medicine purgative in nature.
— Giving blood samples (shocks the system and removes vital nutrients).
— Oil massages.
— Never remain alone (this prevents brooding and dwelling on negative thoughts and feelings).
— Never visit a cemetery (prevents thoughts of death and dying).
— Never take rest under a tree.

LABOUR AND DELIVERY: Natural childbirth at home with only women in attendance is by far the most effective and most psychically easy form of childbirth. Hospitals conjure up images of death and dying and are to be avoided.

Protracted labour is to be avoided — it works a hardship on both mother and child.

Following delivery, the child should be fed nothing but a few drops of honey until the black stool from his bowels is passed out. At this point breast-feeding may begin.

Both during pregnancy and after child-birth the mother should spend her free time reading scriptures and stories of great heroes. She should delight in the joyous achievements of men past and present, creating an atmosphere of joy and gaiety. She should read books about physical culture and postures for her thoughts become part of the child's world, and thus learning of *yoga* will come without difficulty.

Nursing

The milk of the mother's breasts should always be tested before nursing. Pour a few drops into a glass of water. Let the infant nurse only if the milk mixes with the water, not if it sinks, floats, or has a foam or fibrous content. If the mother cannot nurse, fresh cow's milk which has been brought to a boil and allowed to cool should be given.

Foods good for nursing mothers include lentils, kidney beans, cow's milk, clarified butter, goat's milk and rock salt. She should avoid meat, greasy foods and sleeping during the day.

A tea made with cardamom, whole black peppercorns, blackberry bark and licorice root taken morning and evening purifies the milk (boil a half-teaspoon of each in two cups of water until one cup remains.)

If the flow of milk is delayed after the infant passes out the black stool, a mixture of two parts honey and one part clarified butter may be given to the child three times daily.

Mother's milk is the best food for the growing infant, the one designed expressly by nature to suit his own systemic needs. The child should be fed on this vital nectar for the first 12 to 18 months of life. If the mother's milk does not flow or is consistently impure, cow or goat milk should be given instead. It is always best if the milk is of that day's milking. Never boil the same milk more than once, nor allow it to stand on heat after boiling — otherwise the child will suffer from gas.

A baby should never be given canned, bottled or prepared foods. These are already old, difficult to digest and can never replace the vital energy of fresh milk.

A child should never be nursed or given food more than four times daily. Midnight feedings are also to be avoided as they tend to promote digestive disorders later in life.

The mother who is breast-feeding her child should take care always to remain cheerful. The chemicals she produces in her system are transmitted directly to the child through the milk. As a rule, never nurse when angry, tired, sad, anxious, tense, nervous or feverish.

The right breast should always be offered to the child first, then the left.

A mother should stop nursing her child after he reaches 18 months, or as soon as she becomes pregnant with another child.

Nursing can be an exhilarating experience for the new mother, and fulfils deep emotional needs for both her and the newborn. Many of the emotional disturbances of the present generation can be directly linked to bottle-feeding and placing the infant in a separate crib soon after birth.

General Rules for Infant Care

1. Lift the infant carefully. Bones and muscles have not developed fully and permanent damage can result from careless handling. Never drag a baby or toss him into the air.
2. Never terrify or awaken an infant suddenly.
3. Don't force a newborn to sit upright, as hunchback and severe back disorders can result.
4. Always speak sweetly to the child, never in a harsh or angry tone.
5. Protect the infant from strong wind, bright sunlight, glare, bright lights and electric shock.
6. Never leave the child alone.
7. Silken clothes and bedsheets make the infant happiest. Never use synthetic fibres on or near a baby — only silk or cotton.

8. Never allow the baby to be too hot or too cold. Never use an electric fan in hot weather on a child — a palm branch or bamboo hand-held fan works best.
9. Keep an oil lamp burning continuously near the newborn for the first 40 days of life to stimulate pineal gland function and eye coordination.
10. Don't move the baby out of the house for the first four weeks of life.
11. Start solid foods with well-cooked fresh cereals after the first six months.
12. Shave the infant's head after the first year to reduce brain heat and allow full development of mental faculties. This practice also gives stronger hair in adult years.
13. Keep a tub of clay in the infant's room, where he can lie down and play. Use fresh, pure clay and don't be alarmed if he eats a little — it is good for his developing system.
14. Let the child wear little or no clothing during the day so that his skin may breathe fully.
15. Only pure cotton diapers — never paper, nor plastic pants — should be used. Never use toilet paper on the child's anus — wash off with fresh cool water instead.

SPECIAL NOTE: To prolong the infant's life and provide an infallible memory, rub a piece of pure (24-carat) gold on a washed stone each morning while facing East until an amount equal in weight to a grain of rice collects. Mix this with honey and clarified cow's butter and administer daily to the infant for the first six months.

EMOTIONAL DISTURBANCE: A small spot of lamp black on the child's forehead, just above the centre of the eyebrows, diverts the attention of others from his eyes and prevents his receiving anyone's bad sight. If the child does become disturbed and the condition persists, a woman of the household can remove the negative vibrations by passing any of the following three items around the infant's head as the child sleeps. The woman should always meditate first:

1. A stone, which then should be taken outside and thrown on the ground.
2. Seven salt crystals (which should then be thrown in running water).
3. Dried red chilli peppers (which should be thrown in fire).

FOR CRYING: Crying is a natural function caused by an imbalance of body chemicals affecting the liver. Once crying starts, the child should be allowed to express his emotions. However, if his attention can be diverted into some other activity, this is always preferable. No sweets should ever be given anyone who is in a tearful mood — never bribe a crying child with sweets. Sugar stimulates the liver and actually increases the need to cry.

FOR NIGHTMARES: For a child or anyone suffering from nightmares in which deep sighing or groaning sounds are produced, simply remove the sleeper's hands from the chest region and the bad dream will stop.

TO SHAPE THE HEAD: To allow the newborn's head to develop into most beneficial shape, use only a pillow which has been covered with silk and filled with mustard seeds. Mustard seeds adapt to the shape of the skull, and also provide heat to the developing tissues. Mustard oil should also be massaged daily into the top of the child's skull. Only during this period of life can lubrication be directly administered to the brain tissues (the fissures of the skull are still open.)

TO PREVENT COLDS: During the "cold season" an infant should be given one small stamen of saffron, mixed with honey following the same principles outlined in the BLACK PEPPER section. Saffron provides readily usable heat in a form safe for the delicate developing system.

EARLY WARNING: If a child of any age is seen

sucking on his lower lip (that is, drawing it inside his mouth), the parent can be certain that a disease is starting to gain a foothold in the child's system. Stop the child from sucking the lip, and immediately change his nostril to avert disease.

TEETHING: For a small infant, toys made of beeswax provide a safe means of teething, which at the same time will provide both heat and nourishment needed by his system. The wax also has medicinal properties to heal sore gums caused by cutting teeth. Toys made of wood are also helpful.

Fourteen

Why Jewellery For Health?

Every pore of the body is a mechanism for absorbing electrical and magnetic energy into the system. And this energy provides ionic charges, either positive (Cathions) ions or negative (Anions) ions. These ionic charges are directly transferred to the lymphatic fluids, and from there transferred to the blood plasma, which contains a great many conductive chemicals (called electrolytes) in solution. These electrical and magnetic charges promote the natural flow and, according to their nature, affect the operation and development of many systems within the body. It is for this reason that from times immemorial man has been attracted to the wearing of precious gems and ornaments in the form of jewellery.

According to Indian traditional sources, even the villagers wore golden helmets, bracelets and earrings as a matter of course (this is also verified by the accounts of the Greek Menander and the Chinese scholar Phion), as well as many varieties of gems and minerals.

The selection of gems may sometimes do more harm than good, because man is often drawn towards his opposite more strongly than towards that which conforms to his own nature. But one equipped with a real understanding of gems and metals can use his ornamentation as a powerful tool for balancing his psychophysiological system to avoid the needless waste of energy and attain a greater sense of personal security for his own life.

There are nine principal gemstones which may be worn to produce specific effects on the human system. These are ruby, pearl, coral (red), emerald, topaz, diamond, sapphire, zircon and catseye (chrysoberyl). These nine stones correspond to the energy frequencies of the nine planets considered important in the Indian astrological system. Ruby is Sun; pearl, Moon; coral, Mars; emerald, Mercury; topaz, Jupiter; diamond, Venus; sapphire, Saturn; and zircon and catseye respectively for the North and South Nodes of the Moon (called Dragon's Head and Dragon's Tail).

According to the *Rig Veda*, the oldest existing human document currently known, gems and diamonds are the products of the action of intense heat and fire. The quality of creating gems is accorded to Agni, the Lord of Fire, who makes them out of earth. This theory accords with the beliefs of modern mineralogy, where intense heat and tectonic pressure within the earth give rise to the rocks which bear the precious stones.

These gemstones and metals represent the highest crystallization of the ions of elements and elemental compounds. They are formed in the process of purification and concentration of these most essential forms of matter. As such, they have a great potential to absorb, radiate and reflect different frequencies of light. A cut piece of diamond is very much like a pyramid in its ability to concentrate and focus energy.

This connection between fire and gems as explained in the *Vedas* makes it apparent that the body fire as well reacts to these little crystalline transmitters, and the system can absorb the light energy as received and refracted by the gems which are worn. This immediately indicates the possibility of utilizing the refractive powers of the various gems to augment or offset certain energy configurations within the body. According to the *Vedas,* it is the interplay between the elements and the earth's inner fire which converts ordinary chemical substances into gemstones. This too corresponds with contemporary geological speculation (where the various minerals are seen to rise out of a common solution according to the duration of the time the solution is allowed to cool. Rapid cooling creates an undifferentiated mass, while slow cooling allows the different elements to join together according to their own kind and produce large crystalline structures, including the gems).

The *Vedas* contain clear references to the therapeutic use of the gemstones in the 6th Mandala, 19th Sutra, 10th Mantra, where man is advised to wear gems and diamonds to achieve the crystalline fire which has been preserved inside them by the alchemical fire inside the earth.

From these indications it can be readily seen that wearing the proper gemstones and metal can form an important part of the work of synchronizing the system with the energy of planet and cosmos.

Returning momentarily to the archaic roots of the usage of gemstones to change individual energy patterns, Indian mythology calls diamond the *vajra* (thunderbolt) of the King of Gods, Indra. It is Indra who wields the *vajra* to kill the demon of instinct, of base drives. Indra wore the diamond tied to his upper arm, a practice said to give extraordinary power to the hands and complete mastery of the organs of perception and action. In the *Agni Purana,* in the *Mahabharata,* in the *Devi Bhagwat, Garuda Purana* and *Vishnu Dharmotra Purana* and a score of other ancient scriptures can be found clear mention of diamond, ruby, sapphire, emerald and detailed instructions for the usage of each. So the use of gems to modify human energy fields dates back at least 7,000 years according to the recording of Western scholars on the age of these ancient texts. To evolve to this level of understanding, it is logical to assume that the use of gems dates back many millennia earlier. The earliest example of mounted gems from India according to archaeological evidence is a ring from the excavations at Chanu Daro in the Indus River Valley.

Properties of Stones

Indian medical science describes precious stones and metals in terms of five primary qualities:
1. *Ras:* state or effect.
2. *Guna:* particular attributes.
3. *Veerya:* power to interact.
4. *Vipak:* the interaction itself.
5. *Sakti:* the result of the interaction.

These five basic qualities are present in all gems, though their character varies from individual gem to individual gem. Thus some gems have *shakti* (power to produce positive effects) only when powdered, burned and then eaten. Others have effect only from being worn. Those which have the greatest effect when eaten are the least powerful. Those which act when applied as a paste externally have more *shakti*. Those which have power to act merely when worn in small numbers or size have the greatest *shakti*. The nine gems which will be considered in the following pages all fit into this last category.

Colour is an important aspect of the power of gems to work on the human system. Colours are directly related to the three *Gunas: sattva, rajas* and *tamas.* From the same *prakriti* three colours evolve: white (*sattvic*), red (*rajasic*) and black (*tamasic*). The other colours evolve from these basic three, and the colours of the nine primary gems represent specific combinations most useful for human life, as the colours refracted and reflected by these stones have the most powerful concentrated effects.

Different colours of light are the result of different wavelengths of energy. No two human beings need exactly the same wavelengths of energy. To understand the type of energy one needs, one must see the correspondence between the gem colour and the planetary colour. These particular colour frequencies which are found in the nine gems have the power to attract the wavelengths of energy characteristic of the nine planets — be it either directly from the planet, or from the Sun (which is the father of all other planets). By making the proper selection, one can compensate for energy deficiencies in his own system.

Real or Synthetic?

One of the first questions one must ask is this: should I use real gems, or modern synthetics which have the same chemical composition — and apparently the same colour?

First it is necessary to look at the way both types are produced. Natural gemstones are found only at those places on the earth's crust where there has been excessive heat — either from within the Earth itself, or from prolonged exposure to solar radiations. The richest deposits of gems exist within certain well-defined areas which can be termed *solar belts*. One who studies the theory of continental drift finds that most of the rich gem-producing regions were all part of one contiguous mass. The richest areas for gem production have been the Oriental solar belt, South Africa and South America.

Geologists divide rocks into three major classes: igneous (fire-formed), sedimentary (formed by gradual accretion in water) and metamorphic (changed from one kind of rock to another by intense heat and pressure.) With the exception of pearl and coral (both formed by living organism), all the planetary gems were formed by fire, and are to be found in either deposits of igneous or metamorphic rocks. Igneous rocks arose out of a vast, undifferentiated "stew" of molten stone. As the stone gradually cooled in vast underground domes (batholyths and lacolyths), the individual elements began to concentrate themselves together. With the passage of thousands of years, the mineral became more and more concentrated and began to take on crystalline structure, just as sugar or salt dissolved in water begins to crystallize if left undisturbed. With more time, the crystals become more concentrated, larger in form and more perfect. The size, colour and quality of the crystal depend directly on the length of time taken to cool.

Natural gemstones evolved over thousands of years, the end products of a vast complex of gradual differentiation. They formed themselves according to universal and natural laws of deposition and crystallization.

Synthetic gems, on the other hand, are created from already differentiated elements — the reverse of the natural process. Artificial rubies are produced by combining refined aluminium and oxygen in a high-temperature chamber. Chemical dyes are added to create the red colour of the gem. Sapphires are created by the same process, and with the same chemicals, only adding a different dye. These synthetic gems lack all crystalline unity, being merely a rapid and artificially produced accretion. There is the same difference here as rock sugar which has crystallized out of solution into large individual crystals — and rock sugar produced by rapidly melting refined sugar on a stove to produce a large, non-crystalline mass of sugar.

Artificial gems lack the same crystalline coherency which is found in natural gems — and it is this crystalline structure which enables the natural gem to serve as a powerful natural antenna for solar and planetary radiations. Synthetic and glass beads and gems do not possess the same molecular and crystalline structure, and cannot produce the intense concentration of energy radiations. It is only through solar energy that the gems get the crystalline form which absorbs light of its own frequencies and provides it to the body through the skin and paralymphatic glands.

What Stones To Wear?

When selecting gemstones to wear, one should always work with his natal astrological chart — the birth chart. The most important factor to consider is the first house, or ascendant. The ascendant is the most important house in the whole chart, for it is the influence present here which shapes both body and temperament. Here too are determined lifespan, wealth, fame and health. One who wishes to safeguard these essentials of life would do well to wear the stone of the planet which rules his rising sign, as the ascendant is called.

NOTE: The indications in this chapter concern only the rising sign as calculated by sidereal astrology — that science which considers the planets in their actual placement in the constellations in the heavens. Though this is the dominant form of astrology in India, China, Japan and the rest of the Orient, *it is not the astrology generally practised in the United States and Western Europe.* Astrologers in these countries use an artificial zodiac based on the change of seasons, and not the movements of the constellations in the heavens. Western astrology based on the seasons is called Tropical Astrology. The astrology based on the actual placement of the planets and constellations is called either Sidereal Astrology or Constellational Astrology. *Only the rising sign as determined by Sidereal Astrology should be used as the basis of selecting gemstones.* Otherwise one may find himself wearing a stone which, unbeknownst to him, is actually bringing more negative energy into his life.

All gemstones should be perfect, free from flaws, scratches, ridges, mottling, discolouration, roughness, dullness and other imperfections. Wearing an imperfectly formed or coloured stone may also result in attracting more negative energy.

	Rising Sign	Gemstone	Ruling Planet	Metal For Setting	Minimum Weight Required	Week Day to Buy & Get the Setting
1.	Aries	Coral	Mars	Copper Gold or a Mixture of 3 Parts Gold & 4 Parts Copper	6 Carats	Tuesday
2.	Taurus	Diamond	Venus	Silver, White Gold, Platinum	1 ½ Carats	Friday
3.	Gemini	Emerald	Mercury	Gold	3 Carats	Wednesday
4.	Cancer	Pearl	Moon	Silver	2, 4, 6, or 11 Carats	
5.	Leo	Ruby	Sun	Gold or a Mixture of 7 Parts Gold 1 Part Copper	2 ½ Carats	Sunday
6.	Virgo	Emerald	Mercury	Gold	3 Carats	Wednesday
7.	Libra	Diamond	Venus	Silver, White Gold, Platinum	1 ½ Carats	Friday
8.	Scorpio	Coral	Mars	3 Parts Gold 4 Parts Copper	6 Carats	Tuesday
9.	Sagittarius	Yellow Sapphire	Jupiter	Gold	3 Carats	Thursday
10.	Capricorn	Blue Sapphire	Saturn	Iron-Steel or a Mixture of Silver and Iron	5 Carats	Saturday
11.	Aquarius	Blue Sapphire	Saturn	Iron-Steel or a Mixture of Silver & Iron	5 Carats	Saturday
12.	Pisces	Yellow Sapphire	Jupiter	Gold	3 Carats	Thursday

Jupiter is of especial importance in the charts of women, for it is this planet which governs both husband and sons. A weak Jupiter spells late or delayed marriage

— and strong planets opposed to or conjunct with Jupiter also can delay or even prevent marriage and progeny. Women with badly aspected Jupiter should definitely wear topaz. This is especially true if the rising sign is either Gemini or Virgo and Jupiter is either sitting in the same sign with or in the opposite sign from Sun, Saturn or the nodes of the Moon.

How To Wear The Gem

To have effect on the system, the gemstone selected must be placed in a mounting which allows the base of the stone to touch the skin of the wearer. This allows a direct circuit to be established between the wearer and the gem, and insures the free passage of energy from the stone.

Gems mounted in gold, copper or iron should be worn on the left hand; those mounted in silver on the right.

By following these basic principles one can only select stones which will be visually attractive — and serve as potent tools for evolving personal energy.

Fifteen

Semen, Drugs & Youth

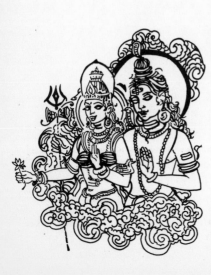

Consciousness does not take birth without semen. Within the germ plasm are to be found all the constituents of the human organism. Semen is the carrier of the genes, archetypes and the collective unconsciousness. Here is the essence of embodied being in microcosmic form.

Semen is the most precious substance in the human body. The components of the reproductive cells and the fluid in which they float are drawn from all organs of the body to the reproductive glands at the command of the pituitary gland in the brain — the controlling agent of both growth and reproduction.

The pituitary and gonads play the active roles in the assembly and dispersal of semen. The pituitary triggers the release of chemicals from the different organs and directs them to the testicles and ovaries. This process happens through the mechanism of gonadotropic hormones.

The essence of the semen is *Ojas*. This marvellous fluid is the life, the vitality, the shine, the glaze of health found on the glowing skin of children. *Ojas,* the viscous fluid in which the germ cells rest, provides semen the strength needed to carry out its journey to fertilize — to unite and become One. Present in both the male and female, *ojas* vitalizes and nurtures the semen before and after conception.

Activities and conditions not in harmony with the life process consume the *ojas.* Disease, chronic tension and indulgence of self-destructive behaviours cause withdrawal of *ojas* from the surface of the body to wash and nurture the vital organs deep within. In such cases, the glaze vanishes and the complexion becomes dry and pallid. The same phenomenon occurs as a result of excessive sexual indulgence.

Loss of semen and *ojas* takes a heavy toll on the body. For *ojas* vitalizes the whole organism — and its loss in quantity spells imbalance and disease. Similarly, the germ cells themselves, drawn as they are from each organ of the body, represent all the chemicals of the organism in their purest and most refined state — and their loss places a strain on the organism.

Normally the system produces an excess of *ojas* (and semen as well in the male)* which is collected and stored in the brain by the pituitary. This excess *ojas* gives vitality to the whole nervous system, and it is for this reason that *yoga* teaches retention and control of semen.

Celibacy

The primary discipline for the control of semen is celibacy. Practice of abstinence teaches retention and control of semen and *ojas,* stabilizes pituitary function and keeps the vibrational rate slow — enabling great concentration and enhancing the ability to meditate.

---

* Here can be found the reason that excessive sexual indulgence is more harmful to males. The masculine system produces new semen with each act of intercourse, while the female is born with a fixed number of germ cells already formed.

Excessive loss of semen and *ojas* pulls these substances from genitals and brain, leaving the mind full of torpor and prey to fantasies and aimless wandering.

For normal life in the world one needs a faster rate of vibration than do the ascetic and renunciate — and thus the necessity of marriage and controlled discharge after one has finished his growth and education. Moderation, however, is always advisable — and celibacy may be indicated when one experiences prolonged states of innervation and depression.

In all cases celibacy is indicated for males before attainment of age 21, and for females before age 18. In both cases *ojas* is vitally needed to support and nurture the still developing system. Any loss can create malformation or improper development of tissues and structures which can affect the individual throughout life.

By adopting a few simple practices one can insure the maximum amount of *ojas* and semen:

1. Men should avoid sour foods and salt as much as possible. Both thin the semen and *ojas*, which must be thick to insure retention. If thin, they can escape through the urinary tract during elimination.
2. Women should avoid sweets and take more salty foods. Salt provides the glaze and glamour of femininity.
3. Men especially should avoid all condiments and seasonings except as necessary. Spices burn semen. Use none in warm weather — and in cold climates, only as necessary.
4. Avoid late-night eating and filling the stomach during meals. Both bring the energy down. Eat no solid food within three to four hours of retiring and avoid tea and hot milk at night.
5. Don't drink alcohol. Alcoholic beverages thin the semen, concentrate energy in the genito-urinary system and arouse sexual feelings and fantasies.
6. Never gaze directly into the eyes of a member of

the opposite sex. Staring causes an energy exchange which can bring energy down. Indian scriptures recommend that men look only at the feet of women.

7. Keep company with the opposite sex only in a well-lighted room. Darkened rooms enhance the capacity to fantasize — especially about sexual matters.

8. Men should wash their legs from knees down in cold water as their last act before going to bed. This concentrates energy away from the genitals, preventing nocturnal emission.

Drugs and Development

The male body devotes most of its energies to growth and development during the first 21 years of life, the female during the first 18. Any stress to the system during these crucial years can permanently alter the formation of body and mind — "as the twig is bent, so grows the branch."

Three octaves of life are encompassed in this span of years during which the organism grows from newborn infant to fully developed youth.

The addition of any external irritants to the system during these years diverts energy from the task of self-development to that of self-preservation — and the maturation process is disturbed, distorted from attaining its full potential.

Semen, kidneys and lungs each play a crucial role in the formation of the youthful body. Semen provides strength, stamina, and health; kidneys clean the blood and filter impurities and poisons from the system; lungs provide oxygen and vital energy (*prana*). These three must be preserved through age 21 to insure a life of good physical and psychological well-being.

Smoking: The lungs regulate the intake of oxygen and *prana*. The role of oxygen in body metabolism is clearly understood. Less comprehended in the West is the energic factor in the atmosphere which is the vitalizing force of all living forms. *Prana* is the name given this animating force which permeates the whole atmosphere, and which we inhale with every breath.

Pranic energy sustains life — indeed, it is the very essence of life. It is *prana* which *yogis* use during prolonged entombment under ground or water to maintain the presence of life in the body. *Prana* maintains and nurtures life. Oxygen can be understood as the gaseous medium through which *prana* is drawn into the body, but *prana* is not oxygen.

Both *prana* and oxygen pass into the system through the myriad network of microscopic capillaries lining the surface of the lungs. The hot smoke from cigarettes, pipes, and cigars has a drying effect on both the capillaries and the thin layer of mucous which coats the lungs and acts a medium to catch foreign substances which have eluded the network of protective devices in the nostrils. This drying effect in turn irritates the nerves and triggers the flow of additional mucous from other parts of the body to counteract the heat and dryness. This new mucous combines with the residues of the smoke to form a dense coating on the beings which significantly reduces their capacity to absorb both oxygen and *prana*. This residue gradually collects in globules causing the muscles of chest and abdomen to contract spasmodically to literally "blow them" out of the system — smoker's cough.

Not only is absorption of energy reduced, but developing joints, tissues and nerves and the action of the digestive system can be seriously impaired by the demand for mucous in the lungs. This fluid is drawn away from the joints (causing a dryness which can lead to arthritis), from the digestive system (which causes digested food to become dry and bound up, decreasing its ability to pass through the intestines — and thus causing constipation and other digestive ailments) and from the head (causing chronic rhinitis and allied conditions).

Another factor to be weighed is the cough itself. Beyond irritating the sensitive tissues of throat and lungs, coughing is not particularly harmful to the organism. To hold back a cough — which smokers often do — one has to act counter to the natural urges of his system, tensing all the muscles used in respiration. This in turn creates an imbalance of the gases which can produce a great many ailments. Coughing is the body's natural mechanism for cleaning mucous-trapped wastes from the lungs. However, one with a chronic cough should never spit out what is coughed up. Spitting out the mucous drains strength from the system. Rather, the coughed-up material should be swallowed, so that the mucous can be recycled into the system. This is especially true for those who are ill — always swallow the cough, or vital strength will be lost and the diseased condition will invariably become worse.

All that has been said about smoking to this point applies to both tobacco and marijuana. In addition to these qualities, marijuana thins the semen, disturbs hormonal balance and by virtue of its intoxicating properties leads frequently to sexual fantasies and behaviour.

For all these reasons one should not smoke anything until his system has fully matured — 21 for men and 18 for women.

Here are some tips for smokers to minimize the damaging effects of their vice:

1. Don't smoke more than one cigarette before the morning bowel movement. Otherwise mucous from the intestines will be needed by the lungs, causing dryness of the colon and constipation.
2. Don't re-light extinguished smokes — they irritate the throat.
3. Drink plenty of liquids — at least a gallon a day — to give adequate moisture to the system.
4. Avoid foods which dry the system. All hot and

spicy items and many sour foods (though not lemon-water and yogurt) have this effect.

5. Take the honey-pepper mixture described in the listing "Pepper" in the Ayurvedic Medicine section first thing every morning, or

6. Take two teaspoons of the skim (*malai*) of milk which has been simmered for an hour or more with a quarter-teaspoon of freshly ground black pepper and — if desired — sugar before breakfast. This counteracts the drying effect of tobacco.

Drinking: Alcohol destroys *ojas,* poisons the kidneys through overstimulation, severely taxes the liver and leads to self-indulgent behaviour. The dangers attendant with drinking have been discussed at length in scores of books, and there is ample evidence that alcohol is poison to the human system.

The body converts part of the alcohol into glucose in the liver, though some alcohol inevitably passes with this sugar into the bloodstream. Alcohol deadens the nerves, while sugar stimulates. This contradictory effect accounts for alcoholic stupor and coma. Hyperstimulation of the liver required for conversion of alcohol to sugar leads to cirrhosis and blood disorders.

Alcohol is also a diuretic, placing a tremendous strain on kidneys and bladder and causing weakness of the urinary tract. Concentration of energy in the genito-urinary system coupled with the drug's disinhibiting effect on the nervous system leads to sensual fantasies and behaviour.

None of these effects is desirable, especially in the developing system — and then only in moderation.

Masturbation: Of all practices in which a youth may indulge, masturbation proves the most harmful to later physical and mental health. *Ojas* is crucially important in the formative years, providing health, endurance and the ability to concentrate. Its loss spells illness, weakness and an aimlessly wandering mind.

In addition, masturbation inevitably arouses guilt

feelings and persecution complexes. Masturbation has rightly been called the "solitary vice" because it is almost inevitably practised is seclusion. One who masturbates fears getting caught, and this leads to feelings of persecution. In addition, once one has done one act which he intuitively knows is wrong, it becomes easier to progress onward to other negative behaviours.

The use of the hands to manipulate the genitals also desensitizes the fingers, for by overcoming natural resistance for the sake of immediate gratification, delicacy of touch is lost.

Sexual energy can be effectively channelled into study and artistic expression — the only means by which full sublimation is possible.

One should avoid all sexually-arousing stimuli — including erotic films, books, artworks, *etc., etc., etc.* In this present age such a task is almost impossible — television, radio, print media and the affectations of the "new" morality continually bombard one with arousing sights and sounds.

When encountering such disturbing stimuli, cast the eyes aside or walk away. Remain centred; keep thoughts on your art, your studies, your God.

Because the human organism is surrounded by an electromagnetic field, one should be very conscious about his habits of standing and sitting. This energy field extends outward from the body roughly as far as one can reach with outstretched arms. The presence of another person within the distance creates a mingling of the two energy fields, which can (and frequently does) lead to sexual play. Also, the presence of another person at a closer distance limits the amount of oxygen available for both persons. As a general practice, one should never sit nearer to another person than the length of his outstretched arms. This creates a capsule of energy around one and enables one to keep calm and centred.

In this domain parents are presented with both a

great challenge and opportunity to guide the growth of a developing being. Overt displays of sensual affection should always be avoided in the presence of children, and the objects presented for their attention carefully selected. This is a great effort, but one which when carried out rightly insures the youth's attainment of his fullest possible potential by keeping his attention centred away from the realm of self-indulgent sensual gratification.

Recognition of the extreme importance of the seminal fluid and germ plasm in maintaining optimal physiological and psychological well-being is not confined to the Indian tradition. Here is a tale from the very wellsprings of the Western Tradition...

A young newlywed once approached the famous Greek sage Socrates for advice. This discussion eventually turned to sex.

"How many times should a man enjoy this pleasure?" asked the youth.

"Once", replied the sage in a calm and matter-of-fact tone.

"Once?" came the astonished reply.

"Very well then, once a year won't cause any harm."

"But sir," pleaded the young man, "I am just married, and to a beautiful and delightful young lady. Surely you don't expect me to have sex but once a year?"

"Very well, then four times a year — taking great care not to allow yourself to fall ill."

"You must be jesting, sir! I am a young man, at the peak of my energy. How can I restrain myself to four contacts a year when I am married to a passionate, amorous woman?"

"All right, then. Have intercourse once a month — and avoid all sudden changes in temperature, keep out of rain and snow, do nothing which taxes the body unduly and eat foods which will provide you strength —"

"But once a month", blurted the groom.

Testily the venerable teacher replied, "Okay — every

night, once before sleeping, once after waking up. But you must do one thing first..."

Delighted the youth exclaimed, "And what thing is that?"

"That you will come with me to the necropolis so that we can have a coffin made to order for your size. Then you may keep it in your home and save your young widow-to-be much worry when your time has come."

The Hindu tradition, fortunately, allows a married man more than one pleasure in his life. Twice monthly will cause no undue loss of vitality to one who is in otherwise good health. More frequent contact will drain energy from mind and body — leaving one more vulnerable to aimless fantasy and disease.